NO HEROIC MEASURES

A DISCUSSION ABOUT THE THIRD ACT OF LIFE

SUSAN OBERG

CONTENTS

From teenage to old age, you are the one constant and unconditional love in my life.
I will love you forever, Craig.

WHAT PEOPLE ARE SAYING ABOUT NO HEROIC MEASURES

Susan Oberg offers a fresh lens through which we can all learn important lessons about aging. It's a beautiful concept to use the art of live theater to tell a story that gets to the heart of what it means to be human. We may not all experience the roller-coaster journey described in No Heroic Measures, but we can all take something important from the stories told in these pages or retold by actors. We all want to take good care of the people we love. Oberg's sketches – in all their reality, grittiness, and humor – can inspire all of us to rethink what it means to age well. They also show the importance of completing an advance directive, like Five Wishes, and talking to your family and doctors about what matters most to you.

Paul Malley, President Aging with Dignity / Five Wishes

All of us will be faced someday with caring for aging parents and family members. Many of us will be placed in the position of Caregiver, Guardian, Conservator, or Power of Attorney. Most of us have no idea what we are walking into as we accept those titles; especially for the people we love.

In this book Sue Oberg shares her personal journey of caring for her aging parents and making decision regarding their life and death. The book is breathtaking, brutally honest, and yet beautifully written through the eyes of a daughter who loved her parents dearly. She writes her story in such a way that you feel she is talking to you as a friend, sharing her experience, her insights and lived advice. She covers topics related to what to expect at a Transitional Care/Skilled Nursing Facility, the effects of serious illnesses on aging parents, the debilitating effects of dementia, and the gut-wrenching pain of making end of life decisions for parents.

During my 40-year career as a Geriatric Nurse Practitioner with a Doctorate in Nursing Practice (DNP) I have seen Sue's story lived, over, and over again, by adult children and siblings who are faced with gut wrenching decisions when caring for their loved ones. The majority of these individuals are walking the journey blindly with nothing and no one to guide them. This book serves as a friend and guide for that journey.

In this book, Sue shares the honest truth, tells it like it is, and sprinkles in some extremely helpful advice. Her warmth and humor make this a truly enjoyable read.

Anyone who has, will be, or is currently caring for aging parents and loved ones should read this book. It is one of the best I have seen!

Dr. Maria Brenny-Fitzpatrick DNP, RN, FNP, GNP

The author, Susan Oberg, has written an honest and heartfelt narrative about her experience caring for her aging parents and has drawn on her many years of theater to provide sketches, both humorous and emotionally powerful. Through these sketches, Ms. Oberg has provided a vehicle to open discussions about the grief, guilt, frustration, and family conflicts that often occur when caring for aging family members. In my years of providing therapy, I have often helped others process their own feelings of loneliness, confusion, and sadness as they tackled the hurdles of the court system, healthcare, and their own family systems. I am pleased to have this resource to recommend in the future.

This book provides an opportunity for others to gather and support each other through challenging times. It can be used by church groups, theaters, support groups, senior organizations, etc. but would also be beneficial for anyone to read on their own as they start their journey as a caregiver. Through her writing, the author opens up about the pain she experienced, the love that helps one get through the challenges as well as grief, and helps you laugh even while confronting heartbreaking and life changing situations. I highly recommend this book to all adult children as well as their aging parents.

Marjorie Law PhD, Licensed Psychologist

INTRODUCTION

Growing up, I was told that nothing was more important than family. When I was faced with the decline of my aging parents, it was natural for me to step in and help them navigate their final act. I wasn't an only child, so I assumed that I would work with my brother and sister, and together, we would make their health and financial decisions. Nothing was too good for Mom and Dad. My family had its ups and downs, but I was convinced that we would pool our mental and physical resources to find the solutions to all the problems in front of us.

So, was it my mom's stroke or my dad's dementia? Was it my dad's anger or his constant demands? It is very difficult to pinpoint when our family imploded, but it did. My sister lived about three hours away, so she did not experience the day-to-day problems. My brother never got along very well with my dad. They were always at odds. When I became conservator, at my brother and father's request, I found myself standing alone with no guidance or understanding of the next steps. And thus, began my journey down a very long and dark road.

As I sat in the courtroom waiting to be sworn in, I had a gut instinct to run. The job of conservator was becoming far more than just being available to my parents. Suddenly, I was facing lawyers, judges, legal forms, and so many laws, it boggled the mind. Imagine sitting on the stand and swearing to the delusions and inability of your father to take care of himself and your mom in a roomful of strangers where the only familiar face is your husband. I stated that Dad was a danger to himself and mom. Was this true? I am afraid it was even more true than I wanted to believe. *This was the worst part, right?* I thought. But this was nothing. I should have realized that it would only get worse. Firmly embedded in my ignorance of the situation, I had this kind of "Walton's World" way of looking at the circumstances in front of me. I thought I could fix it. But what no one tells you is that this is not something you fix. You take that first step, and you start to slide down a mountainside. You try to hang on by grabbing at anything that might break your fall. Each move you make causes you to fall faster and harder.

As the years played over and over in my mind, I kept thinking that there was a reason that I found myself in the position of caregiver. I didn't want to believe that I was sent on this journey for no reason. I knew I had to be present for my parents because no one else was there to take this responsibility. But there had to be more. I wanted to take the most difficult time in my life and make it a positive. Every day when I dissolved in tears, I wished that someone would appear to help me and answer all my questions. But fairy godmothers were nowhere to be found. No one was there to take me step by step through this waking nightmare. I decided I would gather the information and write a journal so I could remember the details and then take this information and hopefully someday figure out a way to pass it on to help someone else. If all I could accomplish is to let someone in the caregivers' world know they are not alone, then it would make some sense.

My idea was to help as many people as I could. I needed a true story with a vehicle to get the information out. Well, since my background is theatre, it only made sense that I would put this into a performance format. The performance elements in this book can be used in a variety of ways. You can utilize as many or few participants as you have available. Best of all, it can be made into a stage production or a virtual production. Maybe you are just looking for a discussion starter with a community of people.

The narrative is to be used with the occasional monologue or sketch included with the story. If the narrative is too long to work within the time allowed, you can make your presentation as long (or as short) as needed. Maybe you just want to pinpoint a specific area for discussion. Find the sketch or monologue that best describes your area of interest or your needs and plan discussion groups around it. Try including professionals. You would be amazed how often you need a lawyer, a psychologist, professional caregivers, financial advisors, and the list goes on. It is time we all discuss what the end of life will look like. We need to let family know how we want them to handle things for us. Trust me when I say a Last Will and Testament is not always enough.

As you read the narrative please know that this is a true story. It comes from a place of love and the hope that we can all develop a better understanding of what our future holds.

1

SENIOR CITIZEN

The other day my husband, Craig, referred to us as middle-aged. I stopped and thought about that for a few minutes. As hard as I tried to join in his fantasy, I knew the likelihood of us living to 126 was pretty, far-fetched. The sudden realization that I am a senior citizen was difficult to digest. I had to wonder, *where did all the years go?* In many ways, I feel like I am still in my forties but that can't be because my children are in their 40s. As I talk to other people in my age group, I find I am not the only one who struggles with the idea of being in the third act of life.

We are at that time where our adult children have left home, Mom and Dad, if still with us, require constant care and help, grandchildren are a joy but bring home the point that our stamina is not what it used to be, and our own health issues are becoming more prevalent. When we get together with friends, the evening is more of an "organ recital" than anything else. A good friend of mine puts a time limit on health complaints at gatherings so people are forced to talk about other things. I want an open and honest discussion on what it is like to be a senior citizen. The third act of life can be difficult to discuss. We need to hear the good, the bad, *and* the funny.

Being a caregiver for parents is not easy. It begins the moment you realize that your parents are not as able to handle their day-to-day life issues and are no longer capable of making all their health decisions. This was an extremely difficult time in my life. My husband and I *lost* three parents in one year. My mom had a massive stroke in 2012, and my dad had dementia for many years. My mother-in-law died from liver cancer. The journey we took would have been so different if we'd had a better understanding of what the future held. As I tell you this story, my hope is that it will somehow help those that are just beginning this difficult struggle.

In hindsight, I realize I would have given a great deal to have a book or a manual on how to take care of my aging parents. It didn't need to be hundreds of pages or include step-by-step instructions. I just needed someone, anyone, to tell me my thoughts and feelings were completely normal. I needed to hear someone say to let go of the guilt and fear and just do the best you can, that it is okay to laugh, and it is okay to cry. You will have those days where you just want to run away. But then you will also experience precious moments that will help you go on after the journey with your parents is complete.

One problem almost every family has is telling Dad he can no longer drive.

Sketch 1: Keys

HONOR YOUR MOTHER

By the time you realize that your life has changed to that of a caregiver, you are in freefall, and you need someone, anyone, to throw you a lifeline. Everything you thought you understood and believed to be true about family has vanished. Along with it goes your confidence and optimism. Your life is a fractured fairy tale that has a big bad wolf on every page.

Mirror, Mirror on the wall

Give me patience, so I don't kill them all!!

Please understand that you won't always feel this way. But if you get to the point where I was, you will begin to question your sanity. You keep telling yourself that you are a capable person, and that you love these people who raised you. I am a mother of three grown children, but nothing prepared me for the years of caring for Mom and Dad.

Everyone knows that at around age 70, we all lose our filters. You know what I mean. As a younger adult, most of us have a kind of "cloaking" device that hides our truest feelings and keeps us from blurting out the complete truth (or at least the truth as we view it).

My mom said when you turn 70, you can say anything you want to, as long as it isn't hurtful. But who makes the decision as to what is or isn't hurtful? Due to the connection you have to your parents, good or bad, they can derail you with what they consider a very innocent statement. Statements that begin with "I've been meaning to tell you" are never good. Conversations prefaced by that short, seemingly innocuous sentence can cause the strongest flight or fight response known to man or woman.

When my mother would approach me with a need to set me straight, I would think, *quick, quick, I need a diversion. What can I say that will distract Mom from what she is about to tell me?*

Mom would say, "Suzie, I have been meaning to tell you ..."

Panic would set in and I would set a diversion in motion, such as, "Mom, do you think Uncle Felix is gay?"

"Suzie! Why would you say such a thing!? Not that there is anything wrong with the gays but why would you say that? Who told you that? Just because he worked a couple years tuning Liberace's piano doesn't mean he is gay. Your uncle was just very musical."

Yup, and before long she would forget what she was "meaning to tell me." Now mind you, this tactic took years to develop. My "topic changer" had to be of great interest to her, not about me, and so shocking that it completely changed the plan of attack. If the topic was about me, it just created ammunition for the next time she was "meaning to tell me."

I truly believe the things our parents tell us are meant to be helpful, or maybe they think they are still taking care of us as they once did. So, we shouldn't flinch when we hear Mom say ... "I am worried about your health." *Insert long pause here.* "It is probably your weight."

Or she might say, "Are you working too hard?" "You look so tired." W*ait for it.* "I suppose it could just be your haircut."

There it is. And before long, you are wishing someone would drag you out back and shoot you. You crawl out the door relieved that you might have a couple days before you are told all the ways you don't quite measure up again. The filter is gone, and you are the target of their new-found verbal freedom.

Sketch 2: Generations

WORTHLESS

W hy are we all so impatient? When did family become too much trouble? We should gather and hold onto every moment we have because you just never know when your life is about to change. Suddenly, with absolutely no preparation, you are looking into Mom's brown eyes in search of some recognition. She is fighting her way through a debilitating stroke, she looks up at you and smiles a crooked smile, and you know that your visit means the world to her. But now she has this quality of a sweet child and all she wants from you is to spend some time with her. Her speech is almost completely gone except for a few sentences. She lights up as you walk through the door and say with a smile, "Sit down! What do you know?" You tell her about the day-to-day activities, show pictures of her great grandchildren and fill up her candy dish. Mom really can't carry her side of the conversation, but that is okay because as you lean over her chair and give her a kiss goodbye, she reaches out to you. You say ... "I love you, Mom." Her automatic response is, "I love you too."

A week before Mom had the stroke, she asked me to come visit. She wanted me to understand that, if anything should happen, she did not want any heroic measures. I was thinking to myself—*Mom, I have heard all this before. I know, I know, I KNOW!* You see I hated talking about losing my mom. I particularly hated the conversations about who received her jewelry. But today was a discussion about how she knew everyone would be able to let her go. Her concern was that **I** would fight her no heroic measures mandate. She was intense, and I could tell this was so important to her. I said, "Mom, I understand."

This one statement created more heartache for me then any one person could withstand. A week later, on November 22nd, I was looking at my mom's blank stare, and I knew that the woman I loved so much was gone forever.

That day, the phone rang around 10:00 a.m. This was not unusual. However, a call from my dad was unheard of. His first words were, "Your Mom won't talk to me."

My first thought was, *well, here we go again.* My parents' relationship had more ups and downs than most marriages. As a child, it was unsettling. You never knew from one day to the next if Mom would be crying or Dad would be putting on his sullen act that he had really perfected over the years. As an adult, it became irritating to the point of being ridiculous. There was one time in particular that I will never forget. My cell rang as my husband and I were doing some Saturday errands. It was Mom. She sounded upset and said, "Well, Dad is leaving me."

I can't tell you the number of times I heard mom crying, saying that their marriage was in trouble. I rolled my eyes at my husband as she told me that my dad was so mad at her that he was leaving.

"What did you do?" I asked.

She responded with a long story about how dad, who was in his 80s at the time, was flirting with all the women in the senior home. She had followed him down the stairs and there he was, talking to Myrna. "Well, I walked right up to them and said, back off! He is my man!" Mom said.

Okay, so, did I doubt dad was strutting around like a big old rooster? Nope! But Mom come on! I didn't say this to her, but I was thinking it. Instead, I said, "Well where is he now?"

"He is standing at the front door. I think he is serious because he has his suitcase, his sleeping bag, and his prune juice."

Trying not to chuckle I replied, "What!? Is he going camping? And prune juice?"

She must not have liked my response because she said, "You know your dad never liked you. He thinks you are worthless!"

Suddenly any part of this that might have been humorous ended in my complete devastation.

Sketch 3: Proud

4

OPINION OR FACT

Have you ever had the wind knocked out of you? No matter how hard you try, you can't talk or breathe. I don't remember much else about that day. But I do know the word worthless never left me again. But back to my dad, and what the phone call was all about.

"Dad, what did you do?" I asked.

And he responded ... "I don't know." His voice was that of a scared child.

"Dad, Mom *won't* talk to you or she *can't* talk to you?"

He mumbled something about not knowing. I told him to call 911. He was terrified and told me that he would wait until I got there.

"I am on my way, Dad. Call now!" I pleaded as I rushed out the door.

When we pulled up to the doors at the senior home, the ambulance and police cars were already there. I ran to the elevators. The minute the doors closed I was mad at myself for not taking the stairs. What is it about elevators in senior facilities? They are so slow I could have run the stairs twice in the time it took to reach the third floor. (No comments please, I am just trying to get my point across.) As I pushed through their front door, Mom was on the gurney and Dad stood leaning against the wall. He looked so small to me. My father was six feet tall but that day, he looked like a small child; he was scared and confused. I went to the gurney to smile at Mom, and to try and reassure her that I was there and that I would make sure everything was okay.

You see, many years ago, when I was a young mother, this woman was my best friend. She was my champion and made herself available at every turn. All three of my children loved their grandma. They adored everything about her—from her lullabies to her chicken and dumplings. The woman that looked back at me now *was not* my mom. There was no recognition. She was vacant and cold. Her stare was suffocating. I told the paramedics that I would ride with them, but as I turned to walk out the door, my dad was standing there with tears rolling down his cheeks. I ran back to him and hugged him. I needed to be with mom, but how do you leave a child alone? At that moment, my husband walked in the door and told me he would get my dad and meet me at the hospital. I was so thankful. I ran to the ambulance.

As I stood in the ER watching them work on my mom, I had never felt so helpless. I knew it was bad when the head nurse put her arm around me. She was telling me to prepare myself. I had an odd response. It was one of anger. *Don't give up on her,* I thought. *Get over there and fix this!* Suddenly, it was like I was struck by lightning and the words "No heroic measures" washed over me.

Later, as she lay in the hospital bed, the neurologist told us it was a stroke. The doctor went into a long description that no one in our family understood or cared about at the time. The next steps needed to be decided. Dad's mind was made up; we were to let her go. His response was so automatic that I felt like I needed to intervene. You need to understand that my dad expected the world to bow to him. I can remember as a young child my dad telling me, "Today it is about me. Someday it will be about you." I never realized how selfish this concept was until years later when I had my own children. So, when my dad wanted to let her die, I couldn't help but wonder if that outcome was for him or for Mom. At the same time, I kept telling myself remember… *no heroic measures.*

I asked the doctor, "If this was your mom, what would you do?"

Her opinion was far different than my dad's. She felt my mom could come back from the stroke. However, it would take time in a skilled nursing facility. And then she said the words that no senior citizen wants to hear—mom would need a feeding tube for a while. My father would not listen. He insisted that we should let her die. The room went silent as everyone tried to digest what my father was saying.

We took dad home, back to where the day began. We got him settled, and we went home ourselves. The day kept replaying itself. I couldn't believe that we were to decide whether my mom lived or died. Did no heroic measures mean she wanted to die no matter what? She was 88, so does that mean you don't try as hard as you would if she was in her 60s? Mom and I had not discussed anything to this degree. No one ever believes that they are going to be faced with this decision.

I needed to see her again. I couldn't wait until morning, so my husband drove me back to the hospital that night. I felt like the answer was there. Somehow my mom would give me a sign. I sat close to her bed watching her sleep. I didn't want to take a chance that I might miss a message no matter how small. Her lips were so dry and cracked. She fluttered her eyes open occasionally but the

Mom I loved was not there. I looked for a nurse to help me wet Mom's lips, but there were too many patients and not enough nurses. I took the swab and tried to help moisten her lips. But because she couldn't swallow, she started coughing. It really scared me. I tried to lift her head off her bed a bit. She settled in again. I sat and wondered if that was my sign. She couldn't even swallow a trickle of water. *Please Mom, please tell me what I should do.*

I returned home with no idea of what was the right thing to do. I just wanted that time back. It was only a week ago. I should have asked more questions. What did she mean by no heroic measures?

The days that followed gave us little insight as to what was right. My dad sat in her room and growled at anyone who came close. The doctor stood before us. Mom was failing, and the decision had to be made. Either we went with the feeding tube or we watched Mom die from starvation. I thought about Mom's life and what was important to her. The first thing that came to my mind was that she was a Registered Nurse. She was extremely proud of this accomplishment. She had great respect for most female doctors. She knew how difficult it was in her day to succeed in a male-driven world. So, the choice was made to trust the woman neurologist because my mom would have trusted her as well. They immediately got her ready to have the feeding tube placed. Dad was beyond furious. His words were sharp and cutting. He snarled and paced in Mom's room.

I followed the gurney taking Mom to surgery. All the time, I was telling the nurse how important this woman was to her family and to please take care of her. I sat in the waiting room, close to the doors that they rushed her through. It was so quiet. No one was there. It was the first time I had a minute to think about the choices that were made. I started to cry uncontrollably as I finally acknowledged the loss of my mom. I promised myself I would fight for the woman that was having the feeding tube placed in her. However, in my heart I knew it wasn't my mom. There were other family members upstairs fussing over my dad, the growling bear sitting in the corner. My only focus was on the woman I feared was fading away.

The procedure went well, and she was up in her room once again. Over the next two days, Mom improved from critical to stable. She still did not appear to know or react to anyone. It was time to move her to a place for rehabilitation in hopes of a recovery. I found the social worker in the hospital to be less than helpful. This was not what I expected. I had worked with social workers in my job and found them to be very caring. This was not the case in this hospital. Maybe she was overworked. However, there was no excuse for her behavior in my opinion. It took a great deal of time and pushing, but finally Mom was moved to a transitional care unit about thirty minutes from my house. It was the facility with the best reputation; it was also very neat, clean, and beautifully decorated. That was when my education began.

This facility had a phenomenal reputation. I had asked many people about their experiences there and read everything I could. As time went on, I learned that even though people have excellent experiences in independent living or assisted living facilities, it does not mean that the transitional care would be the same. As we got Mom settled in her room and the ambulance driver left, the nurse was very present. However, the staff doctor didn't appear until the next day. He made a two-minute visit. He walked in and asked Mom a question. When mom couldn't answer, he said, "Well, okay" and left. He never examined her. I paused a minute in shock, and then I realized he didn't see my mom as a woman who was fighting back from a stroke; instead, she was a piece of furniture that was to be warehoused. We didn't see him again until a month later. I quickly learned that many doctors in senior facilities are not there because of their love of seniors. They are there because it is their only choice.

After his next visit, I followed him out of the room to ask him a few questions. His responses were less than encouraging, and he made me feel as if I had done something wrong. Again, the words "no heroic measures" went through my mind.

I drove Dad to visit every day. He seemed to enjoy his time with Mom, but the silence between them was extremely loud. Dad understood the stroke, but just couldn't process the lack of recognition from Mom. At times he was happy she was there; more often than not, he was angry that I didn't let her go. Every time a new face came to visit, he would comment about how this was not his choice.

His words made me doubt myself. My mom was right not to trust me. I was responsible for this hell she was living. I just didn't have the courage to let her go. That was the story that ran through my mind, each and every day. I was convinced I had failed her. I prayed that God would take her gently home.

Mom, however, did not listen to the comments by my dad. Why? Because she had begun the process of coming back to us.

Sketch 4: Silence 1 or 2

5

DO UNTO OTHERS

Mom was moved to a facility that was deemed "the best" for transitional care, and our journey continued. The neurologist told me not to give up hope. She said Mom could come back to us. My full-time focus was on Mom's recovery. I think back on those days and how I had this false sense of security. Naïve doesn't even begin to describe it.

Care at a senior facility is only as good as the nurses and caregivers on duty on any given day. If you are not present as an advocate for your loved one, they can be forgotten. I began to understand this, two weeks into Mom's care. I arrived early one morning and found my mom struggling to breathe. Her oxygen had been left off and forgotten. Mom was sweating, feverish, and non-responsive. I pushed the button that is supposed to bring nurses running, but nothing happened. No one responded. I ran down the halls searching for help. I found a couple of aides who told me they would be there in a moment. I couldn't make them understand how desperate the situation was. Fear bubbled up inside me and by the time it reached my throat, I found myself playing Shirley MacLaine's role in "Terms of Endearment." Remember when her daughter was dying, and she raised holy hell to get the nurses to react? Well, I played her in the sequel. I like to call it "Tirade in Transitional Care." I may have seemed crazy, but it worked. I had nurses coming from every direction to see what patient had gone off the deep end. It was not a patient. It was me!

After Mom's oxygen was back in place, there was immediate improvement in her breathing. I received the first of many apologies, none of which meant anything, but once again would lull me into a false sense of security. There was always an excuse, but they fell on deaf ears. Their standard "go to" comment was that they were short-handed. I considered that a pretty flimsy defense. When it came to the life and death of *my* Mom, there was no acceptable explanation for inferior care. Period!

My next battle revolved around my efforts to get Mom a bath or a shower. Imagine sitting in a diaper for weeks and not having a bath every day or at the very least, every other day. It took three weeks to make progress on this issue. They had been washing her a little with a washcloth, but comfort was lacking. I was told by her caregivers that she wasn't able to get in a bath or shower. So again, I took matters into my own hands and went to her physical therapist. She told me that a bath and sitting in a shower would be fine for Mom. After three long weeks, Mom had her first bath. I could see the change in her. She visibly relaxed and was able to get some sleep. I insisted that Mom have a bath at least every other day.

One night, I was out with my husband and my father for dinner. I wanted to stop by and check on my mom on our way home. Surprise visits are always a good idea. It was 8:30 p.m. and they were wheeling Mom down the hall in a wheelchair for a bath. Late? Very. But ... better than nothing. However, Mom was only in a shirt with no pants and quite exposed. When I surprised them with my visit, they quickly covered her with a towel.

I followed them as they took her for her bath where they placed her in a big tub. The aide asked if I would stay with her. I had no intention of leaving until I knew she was safely in her bed. As Mom sat in the tub, she fell asleep. I held Mom so she would not slip under the water. Thirty minutes went by, and the caregiver had not returned. By this point, I was up to my shoulders in the water which was getting really cold. My sweater was soaking wet, but if I let go of Mom she would drown. Finally, Mom woke, and I coached her to hang onto the sides of the tub just long enough for me to leave her and reach to push the button in the room that was supposed to alert someone to help us. My first thought was to report the nurse on duty. However, I always worried that they might retaliate against my mom after I left to go home. So, I stayed quiet, and waited until Mom was safe and in her own bed.

I cannot explain the fear and sadness every time I left my mom and went home. My mom had been an outstanding nurse in her day, and this care was unforgivable. I remember when I had my first child, and I was so nervous that I wouldn't be the mom my infant son needed. My mom calmly told me to treat him the way I would want to be treated in the same situation. It seemed so easy. Any time I was in doubt, I remembered those words. It always gave me a sense of strength and love as I raised my three beautiful children. Why couldn't these people treat my mom with the same respect?

Almost every day, I would pick my dad up and bring him to visit Mom. I started to see changes in her. Not a big change but I saw a small light in her that had been extinguished up to this point. I would try and give Mom and Dad time to visit on their own. I would bring my laptop and sit in the dining room and catch up on work. Some days I didn't feel as if I had spent enough time with Mom, so I would come back in the evening. One such night around 6 p.m., I went to check on her. The smell that greeted me at the door told me that Mom was sitting in dirty diapers. She was terribly upset. I saw the tears of frustration running down her face as she tried to get out of her bed. Again, I went to find nurses. Nothing seemed to happen until I got upset. They finally got Mom cleaned up. The aide mentioned sores from the diapers, and I was so appalled at the lack of care, and I told them so. They promised they would change her more often but by this time I had no faith in any of them. Mom was still so upset, and I couldn't settle her down. I found out she had not been fed that day. When I asked the nurse, her response was, "Oh, does she eat?" By this time, the dinner service was over, and the kitchen was closed.

I called my husband, and he brought some soup and I fed her. Mom kept trying to tell me something she was desperate for me to understand. As the nurse walked past the table where we sat, Mom reached out and touched my arm. "Mean," she said.

She told me later that the nurse "slammed doors and yelled." Mom was afraid to go back to her room. We sat with her until late into the night and the nurse went off duty. The next day, I spoke to the new nurse and the social worker. I told them I never wanted last night's nurse to be near my mom again. The aide explained that the nurse really was nice and suggested that I must have caught her on a bad day. She joked about how she teased her for having once worked in a woman's prison. She said the nurse in question could come across as not caring because of that life experience. The shock on my face was enough to make them promise that this nurse would not be in my mom's room again. I wished I had some faith that they would keep their word, but I didn't believe them.

My mom had become so childlike that I felt the need to protect her as much as I did my own children. We had good days and bad days.

So many times, I felt trapped and frightened by the process. But as upsetting as it was for me, it didn't come close to the fear and sadness Mom faced every day. The no heroic measures were meant to prevent this from happening. Doubt clouded my judgement. The story played over and over in my mind. *Mom was right not to trust me. I'm responsible for this hell she is living. Why didn't I just have the courage to let her go?*

It was one thing after another, and I spent most of my time staying close to make sure she got the care that was promised. I had not seen a lot of improvement. At the last doctor's appointment, the neurologist was also surprised at the lack of change. I decided I needed to attend her physical therapy sessions. I asked the facility's therapist if there was something we could do to help the process along. I was hoping Mom could learn to stand and eventually walk. The therapist locked eyes with me and said, "Your mom will never stand or walk again."

The negativity was shocking. But what they didn't know was that I had done my homework, and I knew this to be wrong. They also didn't know my mom. She was not a woman who would give up. My next step was to call Courage Kenny Rehabilitation Institute. I knew it was time to get an independent opinion. Was I pushing too hard? I questioned myself at every corner. Perhaps I was doing this for me. Perhaps I needed to prove something to myself. Sister Kenny's therapist assured me that I was doing the right thing and was not too far off the mark. They were encouraging and saw a good future for Mom. Sister Kenny's therapist made a plan to increase her therapy and created a routine that would encourage her. The facility's therapists were shocked when, in one week's time, Mom was standing and walking with a walker. I will never forget the day my husband and I came around the corner and Mom greeted me with her crooked smile as she took one step toward us. Her progress was slow but determined. Sister Kenny's therapists were so happy with the improvement. They followed her progress, and they continued to help us. They treated Mom like an adult, and as someone who was struggling to come back to her life. Mom responded well to them. We had finally found someone who cared.

The care at the senior facility continued to be lacking. I visited and brought Dad as often as I could. Every illness Mom had was a struggle. We dealt with bladder infections, eye infections, gout, and clogged feeding tubes. We made multiple trips to the ER to get the care that Mom needed.

I began to see little pieces of Mom. She would smile when she saw me. Some days I felt she was very aware, and other days there was no connection. I hung onto every crooked smile and felt blessed each time she directed one towards me.

As Mom and Dad's anniversary was approaching, I saw enough improvement that I thought an anniversary party with family might be good for them. I bought a new outfit for Mom, ordered a small wedding cake, and bought a small bouquet of gardenias. Gardenias had been in my mom's wedding bouquet when they had married 65 years prior. We had pictures of their courtship and lives together on display and champagne and punch for everyone. All their children, grandchildren, and great grandbabies came for the special occasion. It was a wonderful celebration.

A few days after Mom's and Dad's anniversary, I brought Dad to spend the day with Mom. We walked in her room and saw Mom slumped over in the chair, with her nose dripping, and she was feverish. Her bed was unmade and soaked with urine. The smell was very strong in her room. It was dark because the curtains were pulled closed. It was obvious that no one was taking care of her. Again, I went after an aide. Her response was, "Oh, I forgot." "But isn't she listed as DNR."

Mom was very sick. She was refusing food and drink. The change was drastic. I asked if my mom should go to the hospital. I thought she needed an IV for fluids. Their response was your mom is listed as DNR or Do Not Resuscitate. Believe me, no one understood that better than I did. But Mom was suffering, and I knew that she should receive care for comfort. They did little to achieve that. The sheets were changed. We got her in bed, and I asked for the Nurse Practitioner who said she might give her an IV the following day.

After we got her cleaned up and in a fresh bed, the nurses promised me they would watch her and if there were any changes, they would call me. So, I left and took Dad home. After getting Dad settled, I turned around and went back. Something told me she needed me. When I walked in the room, Mom was alone again in the dark. She was not responding, and she sounded as if she was drowning in her own fluids. I knew Mom might die but at the very least I would see that she had comfort and the best of care until she left us. I told the nurses to call 911. I felt as if the cavalry had arrived when the paramedics walked in the door. They were surprised by what they saw and the lack of care and told me so.

They got Mom to the hospital where we soon found out that she had influenza and pneumonia. She was admitted and given antibiotics. The turnaround was significant. Her hospital care was outstanding. The medical staff was kind and compassionate. By the next day, Mom was sitting up and feeling better. The doctor told me that my mom was so dehydrated that the pneumonia didn't even show up on the x-ray. Until they gave her fluids, it was difficult to diagnose the problem.

When do you intervene? When is it comfort and care and when is it going against the DNR? Does anyone really know? I guess we need to follow our instincts. If we truly love the person in question, we will know when to step back and let God take them home. Well, that's what I thought.

Mom never went back to transitional care. I brought her back to live with Dad and got her around the clock care. It certainly wasn't ideal but after three and a half months in a facility considered "the best" it was time. It is impossible to know what is right and what is wrong. So, if you are left with no good choices, I suggest you treat your parents the way you would want to be treated in the same situation. Thanks Mom.

Sketch 5: Isolation

A MOTHER/DAUGHTER MOMENT

It felt good to get Mom back to their apartment. It seemed more normal somehow. However, since the care wasn't sufficient in their independent living facility, we needed to bring in home-care assistance. But, once again, the care was only as good as the nurse on duty. It was hard to find the right match for Mom, but they also needed to be a good match for Dad. Mom expected the nurses to be sharp, crisp, and dedicated. They needed to be just like they were in the days of World War II. I am afraid that was not always the case. My dad liked the company, but never felt they measured up to the care he could give mom. He also was looking for someone to entertain him.

I wound up trying three different home care companies and none were a good match. So, my alternative was to get Mom and Dad moved to assisted living in the same building. This did not work well. Dad was such a bear that the aides avoided him. Let's be honest, no one liked being near him. The next alternative I found was a senior home that was on a smaller scale. At this facility, the care was better for Mom, but Dad couldn't stand the lack of people and entertainment. If you are looking at a private or small care situation, please note that if your parents cannot entertain themselves, private/small home care will not work for them. The food was also less than wonderful. I was constantly amazed at the number of aides who could not cook. Here you had this beautiful private home with a state-of-the-art kitchen and my parents were being served burnt hotdogs. I had to bring them healthy food and add fruit for some nutrition, but even that wasn't sufficient.

Each day my father's personality became even uglier. He was full of anger, and no one could get him to behave. It reminded me of raising a two-year-old which was always the most difficult time for me as a mom. When my children were toddlers, they would stand toe to toe with me, their hands on their hips, and would say, "I do it my own self!!" This was my father to a tee. He did everything but throw himself on the floor and kick and scream. His behavior was hurting Mom's care and improvement. She was finally mobile, and her feeding tube was gone. Her speech was improving but she rarely had a chance to speak; she could only listen to the ramblings of an angry old man. She was walking very well with a walker. I commented on it often.

One day, she broke her silence. "Well, do it or you die," she spouted. We both chuckled, but her comment was not lost on me. I knew I had come very close to losing her.

My mom had so many health issues but was always upbeat, and she was genuinely happy for every visit or outing. One day, I picked Mom up and took her out for the day. It was to be just us girls. I knew this had the potential for upsetting my dad. He never liked the idea that Mom and I were so close. He preferred the focus to be on him. But I wanted Mom to have that special day, and I needed to just be with her.

Our day started at the beauty salon. She got a haircut and a styling. She so enjoyed the special treatment. She could not vocalize it, but her smile spoke volumes. Since her stroke, Mom had lost a great deal of weight. So much, in fact, that her wedding rings no longer fit her. I never really understood Mom and Dad's marriage, but those rings were so important to her. Next, I took her to the jewelry store in hopes of having the rings resized. Her finger was two sizes smaller than it had been before the stroke. We left the rings to be adjusted. Last but not least, we went out for some lunch. Mom was getting tired at this point, so we decided to picnic in the car. It was fast food, but she ate every morsel. We laughed, ate, and enjoyed our time together. I asked her if there was anything else, she wanted to do or if she needed us to pick up anything. She had difficulty expressing what she wanted. So, I went through the list of her favorite things. When I hit upon watermelon, she quickly said, "Yes!" so, I ran into the store and grabbed her a watermelon. She couldn't have been more excited than if I had given her the most expensive gift in the world. We headed back to Mom and Dad's place. I got her out of the car and followed her closely as she made her way with the walker to her room. The improvement in her recovery gave me a good feeling for a short while.

Out of nowhere, my father met me in the hall. He had so many personalities I wasn't sure which face would be greeting me. As he got closer, I realized it was the same person that caused me so much sadness and fear as a child. He snarled at me. He couldn't handle the fact that we had enjoyed a loving Mother and Daughter Day without his inclusion. Their marriage was clouded by mental illness. Dad was never diagnosed but his extreme behavior was bipolar in nature. He put his friendships first and being a husband and father second. His friends meant more to him. He loved to party with them, and anything that got in the way of his immediate gratification was the enemy.

I suppose Dad got married and had kids because his generation was expected to do that. I heard so many stories of his life as a boy. He didn't have the best childhood, but I never saw that as an excuse. I'm not sure if verbal abuse is the correct term or emotional abuse. It was more a matter of silence than verbal lashings. It would hang over the house for weeks at a time. You never knew what caused it. But as a child, you always felt you were somehow not good enough. Unconditional love did not exist. You would do everything possible to get some sort of recognition or love from him. Now, much later in life, that behavior mixed with his dementia and the results were catastrophic.

He spewed venom at me. "You are a bad influence on your mother. You cannot come and see her ever again."

I felt the knife slice away at the last pieces of respect and love I once had for him. I tried to stay calm and not let him see how frightened I was.

"I will continue to visit my mom, but I will leave you alone."

"Don't come and see her again," he responded vehemently.

"You can't stop me," I said, thinking it was funny how young I sounded to myself, like I was six years old again wondering why he hated me so. It made me angry that I gave him that control.

Dad threatened me. "Watch me!" he said.

I walked past him turning my back on him. As I said goodbye to Mom, I anticipated a physical response from Dad, but none happened. I told Mom I loved her. She smiled and responded likewise.

As I headed for the door, Dad followed me and whispered, "I should smother her with a pillow and then kill myself!"

I could not hide my shock. I informed the staff in hopes they would keep a close eye on Mom. These new threats were the beginning of psychiatric wards and locked facilities for him.

My dad tried time and time again to kill me from the inside out. That day, it dawned on me that I didn't need a dad because I had never had a dad. You can't lose what you never had. At least that's what I told myself. I just needed Mom, but I knew she was slipping away.

Sketch 6: Forgiveness

7

THREATS

I returned a couple of days later as promised. This time, I brought Craig with me. My husband had begun to worry about my safety. He suggested I visit only when he could come with me. As we walked in the room, Dad glared at me, got up, and walked away. Mom looked startled by Dad's behavior. I was not. We brought some cookies and Craig cut up some of the watermelon I had bought for mom a few days before on our special day. She loved the visit and the treat but was upset and confused by Dad's bad behavior. Mom became restless and anxious. I didn't know what worried me more. Would Dad's behavior affect Mom's recovery or would Mom side with Dad and tell me to stay away? You see, as a little girl, Mom told me that she would always love Dad more than she loved me. She would explain it by saying, "That's just the way it is!" That visit was a reminder of my childhood. Security was not part of my life when I was young.

I can explain it away now that I am an adult. Perhaps what she meant was that there are two kinds of love. One is for your spouse and the other is for your children. But I could never understand how she could so easily pick one over the other. I fell in love with Craig when I was 16 years old. He is my best friend and the love of my life. But from that love, we created a family. Craig and I together love our children more than life itself. I think if you asked our kids, they would tell you the same.

After days of difficult visits with outbursts and threats, I decided I would follow Dad's request and stay away. My visits caused my mom more anxiety than assistance, so I took a step back for her sake. For the next two months, I was beyond miserable. I wondered every day if Mom was being treated well and if she was happy. One day, I received a call from a friend of my dad's. For me, Jim was an angel on earth. He told me that he was going to take Dad out for breakfast the next day. Jim let me know the time he would be picking Dad up, and how long they would be gone. He didn't tell me directly that this was my chance to see Mom, but I understood that was the reason for his call.

The next day, I drove to the facility and waited in my car. As Dad and Jim pulled away, I jumped out of my car and ran down the hall. It was early, and Mom was a late sleeper. She looked so peaceful and comfortable I didn't have the heart to wake her. I sat and watched her sleep until I was worried Dad would return. Finally, after a few more visits, I just had to see her awake. As I placed my hand on her arm, she opened her eyes and smiled. She was genuinely glad to see me. It was a relief to know I was still welcome in her eyes. Our visits meant the world to me. But this was still darkened by the thought of my dad finding out I had been visiting Mom. I did not know whether part of his behavior was from his dementia or what was a factor of his depression.

Sketch 7: Depression

8

FAMILY CURSE

My father's dementia continued to get worse. His temper and delusions became a threat even to the nurses who helped him. There was one episode when Dad called 911 to tell them he was being held captive by the nurses. That got him a ride to the hospital. He spent time in the psychiatric unit being evaluated by the doctors. After multiple moves from one facility to the next, my brother, now back in the picture, approached me with the idea of me being a conservator for my parents. I had never heard of a conservator, but I assumed it was a fancy name for a guardian. My parents were now in separate facilities. My dad's continued threats had landed him in a locked care center. What I learned over the next two years was that no one wants to be a conservator for a parent. It is a terrible position and people do not understand the heartache unless they, too, have been a conservator.

My brother and I had an agreement that I would handle my parent's care and medical issues and he would see to all the financial pieces. My brother saw himself as a financial guru and was close friends with the trustee my father had chosen. It seemed like the perfect plan. I was relieved to have my brother helping me. However, when you deal with a family member's mental illness or dementia, you never know what is around the corner.

In the beginning, my dad liked the idea probably because he thought he could manipulate me. He wanted to pay me a stipend, but I told him it was not necessary. I mean, why pay *me* when *all* his children were going to work together on his care? It took hours of paperwork and visits to court but suddenly I was the great and powerful conservator. Remember, this was not a job I wanted, but I now had the legal power to "control" my dad. I thought this meant I could keep my mom safe. My brother and dad never got along, and so after a couple weeks, my brother was gone again, along with his promise to handle the financial side of our parent's estate. My sister lived out of town and only came by once in a while. I, however, had signed documents saying I would see to the care of my parents, so I had to be available every day. Honestly, even knowing what I know now, I would still have taken on the responsibility. I wanted to protect my mom. Mom had told me many stories over the years about my dad and his father. They were always "locking horns" over so many things. Years before that, it was my grandfather and his father who fought about everything. Now history and some sort of family curse seemed to have continued. My father and my brother are always at odds. At times, I used to think they enjoyed the arguing, but now it is ugly and never ends well.

Years prior, my brother fought with my parents over some slight he felt when Mom and Dad drove through town and did not stop to see him and his family. I had told Dad to mend fences with my brother. I always said, give him another chance. He is your family. The situation continued and festered for years on both sides. Most recently, my brother was getting married to his second wife and invited everyone except my mom and dad. Dad could not stand the disrespect towards Mom, at least that is what he said, but I knew the anger came from a place of regret. Dad's anger kept growing.

The wedding fell on the same day that Dad was having heart issues and ended up in the hospital for tests. My husband and I met my father there. It took two hours to get to the hospital because of a snowstorm that morning. We spent the day getting the tests Dad needed. All my father could focus on was how upset he was about the wedding. My husband and I did not go to the wedding; instead, we kept an eye on my parents and tried to distract them. We hoped the anger would calm down. At this point, things turned for the worse. My dad insisted that he would disown my brother and take him out of the will. I told Dad that I knew he was angry, but I didn't think this was a good idea. It seemed so final, and I thought he would regret it later. Dad insisted. I thought it was my father's depression and dementia. He even brought in his attorney and trustee of the estate. I did everything I could to finesse the situation. I finally sat down with Dad and said if you disown my brother, I will not be your guardian anymore. So, Dad agreed to let it go, and the storms were quiet for a day or two.

I must admit I am so afraid that this family curse will not die with my dad but will continue somehow in my immediate family. The separation and discord always seemed to be with the men. There is always some distance when your children become adults. That is natural. But when push comes to shove, I would like to believe my children will be there for me and their father.

Sketch 8: Loyalty

9

YES! EVEN YOUR FAMILY

I f you choose not to be present for your parent's final years, that is your decision to make and to live with.

Perhaps you live too far away to be there every day or maybe your relationship with them makes it too difficult to deal with them. Whatever the reason, I ask that you support the sibling that is handling the care of your parents. Do not tell the caregiver what to do. Do not make demands because you think you have a better idea of what the right thing to do is in a situation. Health issues can change every day with the elderly, so you really don't know what the right thing is for either parent at any time unless you are there. Over the years, it takes hours out of every day to see that Mom and Dad are happy and that their healthcare supports them. Before you open your mouth, remember the sacrifice your sibling is making.

If at any time that sibling calls you to update you on a situation, do not think they are asking for you to step in and change the course of action. Do not decide to take matters in your own hands. Be honest with your sibling(s) and do not lie to them so you can make things go your way. When you step away, you forfeit all rights on decision making.

During this journey, I struggled with many things but one of the most shocking was the anger and distrust that my siblings had towards me. I couldn't understand their lack of support. Did they feel guilty because I was there, and they were not? Was it because I was the youngest of the siblings and they thought I could not handle it well? One of the most difficult was the issue of alcohol. I had so much on my plate and had they stopped and realized that when I asked them not to bring liquor to our father, there was a reason. You might say your father is old and nearing the end of his life so he should have whatever he wants at this stage. But what you don't see are the phone calls your sibling receives in the middle of the night because your father has fallen down drunk in the bathroom and won't let anyone help him. You weren't there to witness your father falling as he got out of the shower and could not control his bowels. You didn't feel the heartache and embarrassment for this man as his daughter stepped in to pick him up off the floor because no one was available at the time. Then there are the days that follow where the liquor is not available, and he goes through an angry detox. Your sibling and the nurses will spend hours experiencing verbal abuse as he threatens them.

These were my experiences, and they are not uncommon with aging parents that have had problems with alcohol throughout their lives.

When you know that your parent's journey is coming to an end, be prepared. You need to have a suitcase ready and gas in the car. Whatever you need to get done that will keep you from being at the bedside of your dying Mom or Dad, make sure you have it done. Be ready to leave at a moment's notice. If you do not plan to be there, then let your siblings know. Often a person will fight death if he knows a certain loved one is not in the room. Sometimes they will die when you have left the room. No one knows how the final moments look but think of the family member that sits there and waits for the end to come.

You need to understand that no matter what kind of relationship you had with your siblings growing up, it means nothing when an inheritance is hanging in the balance. I can hear your thoughts as you say, "Well, not our family."

Yes, your family.

As parents get older, they will try to get you to take furniture or other items that are precious to them. Help them get these thoughts written down. Don't just take things because this can be a problem. First, it causes hurt and upset in your family. Second, and most important, your parents may need their furniture depending on the direction their future goes. When you move your parents several times, each facility has different rules on what furniture you can bring. Each move can upset their routine and sense of comfort. If they have some of their own things to surround them, it helps with the transition. If your mom and dad have a few personal items to gift, make sure that their wishes are written down. Jewelry was important to my mom, and she had definite plans, but nothing was in writing. She would tell us over and over how it was to be gifted, but if someone in the family feels they have a right to those certain things, your parent's wishes cannot always be followed.

This was a difficult part of my story to write. As I told you in the beginning, I grew up believing nothing was more important than family. I had no idea that my family would crumble under the stress of our parent's death. It is hard to go on and not have those people in your life. I believe if you plan before you find yourself in this situation, you can better manage the rough terrain. It won't ever be easy, and you cannot plan for every twist and turn, but maybe you will still have a solid relationship with your siblings on the other side of the journey.

After many moves, I was left with my mom who wanted to go to the locked facility with my dad. She would cry every time I visited. She was afraid she would never see him again. Then, there was my dad who was doing whatever he could to manipulate the situation to best suit him. I wanted to keep Mom away from my dad because of his threats against her. But at the time, my mom saw me as keeping them apart and thought I didn't care. I visited her every day, and I would bring treats and presents. She was always sweet and nice, but she was sad without Dad. Finally, my mom's sadness became too much, and I moved Mom to the locked facility to be with my dad. She was beyond happy and so was my dad for a very short while. They put my mom in a separate room. They knew about my dad's threats against her. But the patients in *this* facility had severe dementia or mental illness as did my father. They were good at treating people like my father, but my mom's care was lacking. After a few months, I began to see a real change in mom. She was failing, and I was desperate to change the living situation. I found a place not far away that was big and beautiful. It was the most magnificent senior facility I had seen. And as you know, by this time, I had seen several different properties. The nurses that came to visit Mom instantly adored her as all healthcare people did. I wasn't always completely honest about my dad because I was afraid they wouldn't take him.

The deal was finalized, and Mom and Dad were to move to the new facility. I kept them in separate rooms. This was not Dad's first choice, but as long as he got out of the locked facility, he agreed to almost anything. I felt a huge sense of relief when I put them in their beautiful rooms. Caregivers were everywhere making them feel at home. It took a month for the change because when my parents went into the locked location, they had to give up all their furniture that my sister and brother now had at their houses. We had to buy all new furniture. We bought nice furniture, but we had to put each piece together ourselves with those awful do-it-yourself instructions. It took many days to get the apartment to a level that made it feel like a home. Craig worked long hours putting everything together. We shopped for beds, dressers, dishes, etc.

The minute my mom moved in the new place, I saw her mood and health improve. She was happy. She was using her walker and going to meals and even made friends. My dad was happy too. It was a new place, and he always liked being the new kid and making friends.

As Dad's happiness faded, and it always did, the dementia became more of an issue, thus so did every part of caring for him. One of the biggest problems was his medication. Dad's paranoia became a definite factor. Somehow his meds were seen as the doctors not caring and just wanting his money. He didn't need his pills.

Sketch 9: The Pillbox

10

SNAPPED

As always, a drink was the only thing that made life worthwhile for Dad. Whether it was gin, bourbon, or wine, Dad needed it every day. I knew his doctors didn't want him to mix booze with his meds, but convincing Dad or other family members of that was impossible. Family would arrive with bottles of booze. My dad would see them as his friends, and I became the enemy. He would drink with them, and I would get the call at night when he became violent with nursing staff. Nothing I could say would make family members see his problem as alcoholism. He had been an alcoholic for as long as I could remember. Why couldn't my siblings see that? They grew up in the same family that I did.

Balancing all this along with my mom's care was a nightmare. In the back of my mind was always the fear that he might take Mom's life and his own. How do I go home every night and wonder if my parents would be alive the next day?

I had so much anger built up toward my siblings for their lack of support that I decided I would take the money offered by my father to be his conservator. I didn't need the money, and in the beginning, before my siblings walked away from me, I had no intention of accepting money to be conservator of my parents.

But one day, after cleaning up the mess from a day of them drinking with my dad, I snapped. I called the trustee and told him I had changed my mind and wanted to be paid for my time. Deep inside, I was hoping my sister and brother might realize their bad behavior if it affected them financially. But, instead, they put a new stringent set of rules and stipulations on the stipend for caring for Mom and Dad. They wanted reports, dates, times, etc. It took hours of my time. My siblings didn't believe the hours I declared as time spent with Mom and Dad. In fact, they said I needed to stop visiting so much. I found that to be rather comical. What they didn't see was if they would do their part then I wouldn't be carrying the entire load. The money was minimal, but they saw me as a person taking their inheritance, and the distance between us grew.

Sketch 10: Emotional Abuse

11

HOSPICE MEANS WHAT?

The arguments with my father were ugly, and Dad's breakdowns were so bad that some days I feared for my safety. We tried different meds to help with his mental illness, but pills only work if you take them. My dad didn't believe in medication. He fought them at every step and told me he just wanted to die.

Mom's decline was slow, and I spent so much time with her that I guess I didn't see the end approaching. It was probably more that I didn't want to see it or her discomfort. I finally had her in a wonderful place. The nurses adored her and treated her very well. They also understood my dad and removed Mom from the bitterness as often as they could. They would tell Dad they needed to take her to a therapy appointment but instead would take her for an ice cream cone at a little store at the facility. My mom was always a big fan of ice cream cones.

Mom suffered with congestive heart failure, kidney failure, and gout. There were days when her feet hurt so much from the gout that she couldn't even stand. If you removed her sock, she would wince and groan with the pain. I took her to so many doctors. Understand that

gout by itself is very controllable, but at the time, there was no treatment for Mom. She had kidney failure and the medicine to alleviate
her gout would cause her kidneys to shut down. Every so often she
would have a round of steroids and that would help for a while. But
then it grew like fungus on her hands and feet. She never
complained about her hands, but I could tell she was in agony with
her feet. The cauliflower-looking disease distorted her hands and
even lifted her fingernails. I learned that a stroke can sometimes
affect the part of the brain that is the pain center for different parts
of the body. As a result, the pain did not transfer from her hands. I
was so thankful for that one blessing.

At our last visit to the clinic, Mom's doctor checked her blood to see
how things were progressing. The news was not good. I trusted this
doctor completely. She had not been just our physician, but she was
also a friend. That night, she called and, as gently as she could, told
me it might be time for hospice. She said Mom's kidneys were failing. I knew that was the right thing. But it was nice to have someone
stand with me on the decision. We had been able to have three more
years with Mom since the stroke. She saw weddings and, in fact,
walked down the aisle at my daughter's wedding. She had welcomed
two more great grandchildren into the family. She had birthday
parties and anniversary parties. She spent time with all her children,
grandchildren, and great grandchildren during those years. If she
could, what would she say? Was she thankful for the extra time? Was
she grateful that I fought for her? Did she finally see my worth? I
will never have the answers to those questions. I know that I did the
best I could, but it wasn't over yet. Now it was time for the final
chapter. Nothing was more difficult than the days that followed.

Our doctor took care of the plans for hospice, and my phone was
ringing the next morning. We planned to meet in private and discuss
the very best care for Mom. There were so many misconceptions
about what hospice was going to offer. I thought they would take

care of mom day and night. This was not so. They were available by phone to increase the meds needed and visit once or twice a week. My dad thought that it was finally over. He assumed they would give her a huge amount of drugs and then she would pass away in her sleep. He was furious when they would not follow his wishes. He became sullen and impossible to handle. He was angry once again. He glared at me and said, "You want her to suffer don't you."

He became so vicious that social workers, doctors, nurses, pastors, and hospice care could not control him. That is when he took it one step too far. He told the caregivers that he was going to kill mom and himself and end the suffering. Well, with laws being the way they are, they had to remove Dad. They gave him every chance to recant his threat, but he refused. The ambulance showed up, and they were going to remove him. If this was not bad enough, I needed to sign the papers having him removed and placed in psychiatric care. This was not the first time he had been placed in this facility.

Couldn't he see past his narcissistic personality long enough to realize Mom needed him? No.

It was just as he told me when I was a small child. It was all about him. I had to choose between my mom's safety and my Dad. Mom was in bed by this time and not very aware of her surroundings. How could I take a chance that he might carry out his threats? I signed the papers.

I stood in the doorway of their apartment as they took my father away in restraints. He hollered all the way to the ambulance. I wanted to run and hide. I wanted to be anywhere but there. But I had promised I would see this to the end, and I would not leave her now.

Sketch 11: The Conservator

12

I TOLD HER SHE COULD GO

I turned and walked into the bedroom where she slept. Her breathing was labored. It brought me back to the night she had pneumonia. She sounded like she was drowning. The nurses assured me that she was peaceful. They said it sounded a lot worse than it was. That made no sense to me. She was dying. How could it be any worse?! I sat beside her and talked to her. I told her how much I loved her, but she had already begun her journey to the other side. I wondered what I could do to make it easier for her. The nurses came to change her and make her comfortable. I stepped out of the room for that moment. The hospice nurse asked me if I had told her it was okay to leave. I hadn't said those words yet because up until this time I hadn't told her these people helping her were with hospice. The nurse said Mom needed to hear it from me that it was okay to leave. As much as I wanted more time with her, I wanted her to find peace even more. So, I went in her room after they made her clean and comfortable. Again, I told her how much I loved her. I explained that we had done everything we could. I told her we would all be okay and that she could go. I suggested she find her brothers and her dad and mom. I wanted her to find those who had gone on before her. I sat by her bed and prayed to God that he would take her gently home and to please keep her safe. But in my heart, I knew she would not let go until she heard those words from Dad.

Love is funny, isn't it? Here is this man who made her miserable and sad so many times and yet when push came to shove, that same man was her comfort and safety. I knew there was nothing I could say to release her from this pain and sickness.

Maybe I could convince the staff at the home to let Dad see her. I decided to place the blame on myself for his behavior. I told them that I upset him that day. If you ask me now why I did this, I cannot really explain it. I guess we had come so far, and I still needed to protect Mom. Dad was allowed to visit Mom but only with supervision. He was staying at my brother's house. My brother had gone to the hospital where they had taken Dad after his threat to hurt Mom. They had a space for Dad in an excellent psychiatric unit, but my brother didn't want him to be placed in a locked facility. Of course, my brother had been gone from their lives for over a year, so he had no idea how bad Dad had become. My brother told me they had no room for Dad in the hospital, and he would bring him to his house. I had to agree to it because I was the conservator. So, not having the full story and just being exhausted, I agreed to the plan. The doctor that wanted to admit Dad later got me on the phone to tell me that my brother had lied, and that they indeed had room in another hospital for Dad. The doctor also felt that the hospital was the best thing for Dad. By this time, the plan had been put in motion and Dad had been told he could go to my brother's house.

If you had asked me many years before, I would have said that my brother would have stood by me. Everyone thinks their family will work together when times get difficult. But that is not always the case. When it comes to a parent's death and a potential inheritance, all bets are off. It would have been so much easier to run and never turn back. But loving Mom, the good and the bad, my heart told me to stay. I sat with her for hours. As the wait went on, Dad did spend some time alone with Mom, but I kept a watchful eye. My husband, sister, and I stayed the night as the time grew near. I had never felt such exhaustion. Craig sang hymns to her for hours. She loved hymns, and he remembered.

We went home for a short while to shower and change the next morning. I even slept for an hour. That was long enough though, and I needed to go back. As I was walking out the door, I stopped and decided to grab the music box. It was a wooden music box that Mom had given me many years before. It had been hers for years. When I arrived, some of the family members were in the living room with Dad. I took this time to sit with Mom in her bedroom and played her music box. Her breathing was slow. At times, she would go 30-40 seconds without taking a breath. The nurses came in and out to check on her and give her morphine to keep her comfortable. The music box played on. She seemed restless for a minute, and I asked my son to get the nurse. The family gathered in her room. Suddenly, she sat up in bed and opened her eyes. I told Mom I loved her, and with my sister on one side and me on the other, she died.

There were so many tears, and at times, I had no control. I cried for the loss of my mom. I cried for the loss of my family and I cried for my dad sitting alone in the living room. Did he sit there because he was afraid? Did he sit there because he didn't understand the finality? Or was my dad just relieved she was gone? I can never say with certainty, but I do know a piece of me died that day. The piece that loved family no matter what they said or did. The pain was so horrific that I decided to never let myself be hurt by any of them again.

Sketch 12: Grief

13

BIRDS OF A FEATHER

My Aunt Sarah is without a doubt my favorite relative. She is my mom's youngest sister. When my mom's health declined, and she became weaker, Sarah took over as my champion and supporter. I am not sure if I would have survived without her. I didn't tell her everything I went through because she had immense sorrow in her own life. It hadn't been that long since she had lost her son, Andy, to pancreatic cancer. Andy was a wonderful young man —only in his 40's—when he died. As a parent, I can't even imagine the grief she experienced and continues to live with every day.

Sarah wrote to me multiple times as we prepared the memorial service for Mom. She was full of great advice, but one thing she said was a complete game changer for me. Sarah told me to be open and look for signs from Mom. She said that Mom might send me a sign and that it would be very reassuring at some really difficult moments. I didn't think much about it until the day of the memorial service. I had been working all week preparing for the funeral. It was my last gift to my mom, so I needed the service to be perfect. It is odd, but planning a funeral is almost as work intensive as planning a wedding. The pastor, the church, the food, the music, the pictures were all the same. Of course, there was no cake but being from the Midwest, there were cookies and bars.

That morning, before my husband and I left for the service, I felt myself coming apart at the seams. I had been so wrapped up in the plans that I hadn't had a chance to truly grieve. I felt it leaking out of every pore that sad morning. As I cried, my husband, Craig, came up and put his arms around me. When I cried, it always made it worse when someone was nice to me. Craig knew to give me space at these times. But I also think he knew that no amount of time or space would hold me together that day. As I sobbed in his arms, I kept saying if I just had a sign from Mom that she was okay. I tried to explain through the tears what I meant. Suddenly, the tears stopped as fast as they had started. There, sitting on my deck was a beautiful bird called the Flycatcher. I was frozen in disbelief. My mom and I were avid birdwatchers. I am nowhere near the expert she was. Craig and I had lived in our home for 11 years. In all that time, I had never seen a Flycatcher. I knew this because it was my mom's favorite bird, and I always looked for one.

When I was a little girl, I can remember my mom pointing out a flycatcher as if it were the perfect gift placed in front of us by God. We watched with great reverence. Then the bird disappeared as fast as it had come. I always understood the perfection of the moment and felt as if I had been so lucky to see this feathered creature with a top notch adorning his head.

I pointed to the bird on the deck and Craig asked me what it was. I said, "It's Mom's Flycatcher." However, this bird was absolutely the most beautiful Flycatcher ever. He had a bright yellow breast surrounded by beautiful brown feathers. He stopped, looked at Craig and me, and flew off. Craig smiled and said, "Well, there's your sign. Your mom is okay." We never saw that bird again. Some people would call it just a coincidence. But I knew better.

Later in the month, I was talking to my daughter, Beth. She was having a tough time and missing her grandma. I told her my story and told her to be open to signs as Sarah had told me to do. Beth's sadness meant a trip to Target to peruse the aisles. It sounds odd to some, but to my daughter, shopping at Target is the best therapy.

So, she and her daughter, Lilly, went to her favorite place. After an hour or so, Beth decided it was time to get Lilly home. They checked out with their bounty of things that they just "could not live without" and headed out the door. Please note that this Target was in the middle of Minneapolis. There, sitting by the door, was a flock of ducks. Now this may not be a big deal to some people, but Mom took care of my kids often when they were young and when she rocked them to sleep, she would sing "Six Fat Ducks." My mom was so well known for this song that we even played it at her funeral. When Beth first saw the ducks, she was startled. That was when she stopped and counted. They were six of the plumpest, sassiest ducks you have ever seen. There would be no better way for my mom to reassure one of her grandchildren but with six fat ducks.

I thought about Mom often in the weeks that followed. I felt so empty and lost. Everyone had gone back to their lives, but I felt stuck in a world that was cold and lonely. I tried to comfort myself by remembering the Flycatcher. I got out a bird book that Mom had given me. I wanted to know more about this bird. I looked at all the pictures of the different species. The beautiful bird that we had seen that day was not the typical Flycatcher I knew. He was different because he was native to Arizona, and we lived in the Midwest. Again, I smiled as I thought about the bird, I saw that Friday.

As the days passed, there were other times when I heard or saw something that reminded me of Mom. I never felt sadness but instead I just knew that Mom was close and keeping an eye on all of us. Birds continued to visit my feeders. We have Chick-a-dees, Cardinals, Nuthatches, Orioles, and the list goes on. Never once did the Flycatcher return.

Sketch 13: Lilly Mae

14

FOR BETTER OR FOR WORSE

I have decided that you can never escape who you are at your very core. Each birthday, you become more and more of your true nature. Mom was, at her core, a gentle spirit. Dad was the complete opposite. I watched my mom die with dignity and grace. I was with her as she took her last breath. My dad on the other hand was fighting, biting, and scratching as he came to the end of his life. He trusted no one and loved no one more than himself. And even though his nature was caustic, my heart still hurt to see him die in pain and misery.

It took sixty years, but I finally realized that there was nothing I could have done to create a real father-daughter relationship. The time was up. I resigned myself to move forward knowing from my first memory, that I was never good enough for my dad. No one would ever believe that Dad suffered from a mental illness unless you were part of the immediate family. He was a master at charming people. I guess that is why he has always been a true salesman. But just as quickly as you were his friend and in his good graces, he could change in the blink of an eye. Unconditional love did not exist in his world.

All I can do is try to do and be better. I know that the love I have for my children is so strong that the English language does not have an adjective to describe it. I am so incredibly proud of each of them for so many different reasons. They are intelligent, compassionate, and self-sufficient people. I know I have not been the perfect parent. All I can hope for is that when I leave this world, my children know they were genuinely loved and that my last thought was of them and their father.

My dad's mental illness took apart any relationship I had with my brother and sister. Brick by brick it had been dismantled until all that was left was dust and rubble. It was difficult growing up in this family. I thought as I became an adult and had my own family, that I would heal and move on. I guess we all wear our childhood like a coat. It either keeps us warm or you freeze to death.

The feeling of loss and change is crippling as you go through the journey of watching your parent's age. As they become completely dependent on you, it can affect every part of your life. So many people will say to you, "make sure you are taking care of yourself." There is so much data out there regarding the effect of stress on caregivers. It is natural for family and friends to be concerned about you. However, how does one take care of themselves when they are working full-time and at the same time, spending every spare second taking care of their parents? To take a day or even an hour for yourself does nothing to help the feeling of exhaustion. As much as there is the need to get away, you can't stand the feeling of leaving your parents alone. What if something were to happen? What if the day you don't visit is the day they die? What if they die alone? When you have a parent, who cannot speak for themselves, they rely on you to get their feelings across. Even the best medical staff can't always decipher their patient's needs as well as a daughter.

As this battle continued, I noticed myself coming apart. My health was not good. My emotions ran high all the time. It affected everything and everyone in my life. The one big surprise was the effect it had on my marriage. Most people would assume that it would affect your relationships, but I didn't see it coming. I thought we were different. We had been married for 40 years. Craig and I were each other's best friends. It was truly a miracle that we found each other at such a young age. I had never seen an example of a strong marriage except for on TV. My examples were the Walton's and the Ingalls. This was not exactly a standard that would be easy to live up to at any time. The only example I had was fiction. Yet, we found our way. We were married so young in today's terms. I was only 19 years old, and he was 21. Craig loved me unconditionally. I was crazy about him. It was an incredible feeling to be loved so completely. This is not to say we didn't have a lot of growing up to do, but what we had was always worth fighting for. The only problem we had was his mother. She did not like me or the idea of us. She considered me to be from the wealthy side of town. She told Craig he would never be able to make me happy. Most girls would have walked away from the treatment I received, but I recognized it and saw parts of it as being pretty familiar to what I had experienced in my own family. So, I took the abuse and stood strong against the insults and cold behavior.

About two years into my parent's health struggle, Craig's mom needed our help. We moved her to a facility just 10 minutes from our home. That facility was well known for its caring staff. It was not an easy move for my mother-in-law, and she let everyone within earshot know it. I was afraid that she would pick up where we left off so many years before. However, her health was such that she didn't have the desire to fight with me anymore. We would actually spend pleasant time together and I visited often. She made two good friends at her new home and the staff adored her. They would tell Craig that his mom was so funny. To which he would reply, "My mom?" I would do anything for Craig. If that meant moving his mom closer to us, then that is what we would do. How could I say no? He helped me all the time with my parents, so I would do the same for him.

Craig's dad had passed away several years before from Parkinson's disease. He was a good man with a kind and compassionate heart. I recall one time when we were left alone while Craig and his mom went out to run errands. Craig's dad and I were sitting out in the yard on a sunny day. Out of nowhere, he started talking about Doris, Craig's mom. He tried to explain her upbringing. Her parents were not the warm and fuzzy kind of people. I had heard this from Craig before, but this was new hearing it from Craig's dad himself. Suddenly, I realized that I was not the only one that saw her bad behavior. It was the same language used as an explanation or an excuse for my father's behavior. I appreciated him reaching out to me, but I did not see her childhood as being a valid excuse for her poor treatment of me and sometimes, our children.

Once we had Craig's mom all settled, her care went very well. It continued to be an education in healthcare, but for the most part we got through it. Now Craig and I were juggling two jobs. Each averaging fifty hours a week and three parents with constant needs. When we did have time together, we discussed things such as adult diapers, walkers, electric scooters, etc. I learned that we deal with stress and grief very differently. I needed someone to talk to about all my heartache. At the time, Craig would rather have had someone shove a hot poker in his eye than talk about his feelings. Most people probably would think, *well, that is the difference between men and women.* But up until this time, we had talked about everything.

Remember, we were best friends. I knew our marriage was changing, but who had time to address that?

The firm foundation that had been mine was crumbling, and the more I tried to talk to Craig, the worse it became. I went to a psychologist in hopes of getting some help. But once a week, she would rip the band-aid off the hurt, and I would go home exhausted and feeling worse. She was not the psychologist for me. I knew there were many good psychologists out there, but exhaustion prevented me from continuing the search.

My husband, being a pharmacist, wanted me to try medication. I began having panic attacks, and I couldn't sleep at night. With no warning, I would feel as though my heart was jumping out of my chest, with my breathing becoming fast. These panic attacks would end with me being afraid I was going to have a heart attack and I would dissolve into tears. Not exactly the girl Craig had married. But he wasn't the man I married either. I needed him and felt him being very distant. The more distance, the greater the panic. It was an ugly cycle. Craig buried himself in work and the combination of our stress started to pull us apart. I finally started anti-anxiety drugs. The doctor that helped me with my mom was also my doctor. She knew me well and saw that I was struggling. She suggested medication for my depression and anxiety. The medication worried me because I had a big job that took a lot of time and I had to "be on my game." But I was soon diagnosed with PTSD and I started medication. It was a small dose. In fact, it was not even a full dose, but it was enough to help me get my feet back under me.

While visiting the family doctor, it was suggested that I get a flu shot because I was a caregiver. I had the first flu shot I'd had since I was pregnant with our first son over 36 years prior. I know you are not supposed to get sick from the flu vaccine, but I crashed and burned. I was so sick with fever, congestion, vomiting, and … well, you get the picture. I was in and out of the ER for two weeks with some strange symptoms. At that time, Craig was about to leave for a business trip where he would be gone for three nights and four days. We had done this many times before because it was part of his job. However, I was so sick I was convinced that he would cancel the trip and stay home and take care of me. He was not a presenter. It was more an observational trip, so I knew that skipping it was something he could do. We waited to see if I would improve, but each day was worse than the day before. He frequently asked me if I was better. When I replied that I wasn't, he would not respond. Perhaps it was grief over his mother's failing health, or maybe he needed time to escape reality. Finally, on the morning he was to leave, in a panic, I asked if he would stay home with me. He was angry and acting differently than the man I knew.

He left.

As the door closed, I felt a shift in my world. Was this his fault or was it mine? This was no one's fault. It was just a very sad and difficult time. Months followed and we didn't talk about much, we just plodded on, one foot in front of the other. This was not the first time (or the last) that we were separated by grief and exhaustion.

The reason I tell you all this is because I have learned that you need to have an advocate when you are on this journey. This needs to be a person who is ready to hear your thoughts and will be there for you no matter what. You need a sounding board. Find someone that is not as close to the grief as you are. When you follow your aging parents so far down the rabbit hole, you need someone to be your voice of reason. This person needs to help you see what is right for your parents without sacrificing yourself or your marriage.

Sketch 14: Marriage

15

A DAUGHTER NOT SEEN

The time had come for my dad to begin his journey to the next life. The doctors said his bladder cancer was back. Dad struggled with reality. Between his dementia and the pain medication, his personalities appeared suddenly and disappeared just as quickly.

As I entered the elevator of the hospital, my heart started to pound. I told myself that I had this. I could do this. I argued with myself. *Do I continue to his room or do I turn and run?* My head told me to get in the car and stay as far away as possible, but my heart forced my feet forward.

I came around the corner and a nurse was there with him. I waited in the hall because she was changing his diaper. This alone was more than I could believe. The man I knew wore many hats of independence. He never wanted help or support because to ask for help was a sign of weakness. He would never let anyone see that side of him. This would make him vulnerable, and he couldn't let that happen.

The nurse opened the door and welcomed me in. Dad saw me and smiled and said, "Hello Sweetie." He seemed really happy to see me.

He wanted to hear all the news. I began to let my guard down and enjoyed a moment with my dad. But, as our conversation continued, he started to ask me questions that made no sense. It was then that I realized that he thought he was talking to my sister. He adored her. You could see it in his eyes. I didn't want to break the spell because just for a moment I could imagine what it was like to be loved by my father. I didn't correct him because he needed to believe my sister was there with him. I was so tired of explaining my sibling's absence to my parents. I am nothing if not a master at making excuses.

His lunch arrived and he seemed interested but just sat looking at the tray. I kept talking, cut a soggy grilled cheese in half, and put it in his hand, all the while commenting on how good it looked. He began to eat the sandwich and I slipped a spoonful of lukewarm soup into his mouth. Before long, he rejected my help. I could feel his restlessness coming back. This was always a cue that his anger was close to the surface. He took the spoon from me as if he was going to feed himself. As I started to back away, he put the spoon in his apple juice. I saw the confusion cross his face. *Do I try to help again or stay back?*

The nurse interrupted my thoughts. He needed his meds and I saw this as time for me to leave. I told him I would be back. However, every time I walked out the door I wondered if this would be the last time, I would see him. In a guarded place of my heart, I prayed I would get that call saying he had passed away in his sleep.

I have spent most of my life trying to fix things and make the people I love happy. But I knew there was nothing I could do to fix this. This fact sent me back to an ugly place to where, once again, I am the worthless child that never quite measures up to the goals my dad had for me. I walked down the hall to the elevator and nausea washed over me. I didn't know if it was sadness or fear.

A few nights later, I got a call saying that Dad had a meltdown and Haldol (by syringe) was needed to control him. What does someone do when they receive that call? My gut told me to go and sit with him. But as hard as it was to face, I knew he didn't want me there. I walked around the house trying to keep myself busy. My husband was traveling for work and the quiet and the dark was almost more than I could stand. My kids were all busy with their own lives and I didn't know if they wanted to know how bad things were. I wished I could call them, but I don't want to put this on them. Bed seemed like the only escape. I hoped I could sleep to block out the crazy for a few hours. I was so deep in thought that I didn't see the warm brown eyes watching me until my Golden Retriever's wet nose brushed against my hand. My best friend was reminding me that I was not alone.

I do not know where the survival instinct came from, but it finally set in and I told my brother and sister I would not be the conservator for my father anymore. The way I saw it was that I only became conservator to keep my mom safe. But now that she had passed, I decided that for my health and my marriage, I would back away. It was time for one of my siblings to take this responsibility over. After much discussion, my brother's new wife took over the job of conservator. It took one court appearance, and the final decision was no longer mine. What a relief. I thought it would be better. But at this point, it changed nothing.

As I watched my dad die, many memories would surface; some good and some not so good. Actually, one of my better memories happened only a few weeks before. I had been to visit my Dad and I knew his 91st birthday was the next week. I asked him if there was anything he wanted. He usually would tell me nothing, but this time, he said he wanted a cake and a rare T-bone steak. I guessed that would be easy enough. When I asked him if he wanted his usual

German Chocolate Cake, he said no. He wanted a cake made of doughnuts. I laughed and asked him what kind of doughnuts. He didn't care. So, I went off to a local bakery and told the people behind the counter about this cake that needed to be made of doughnuts. Much to my surprise, they created a cake of three dozen glazed doughnuts that made the numbers 91. I grabbed some candles, and his cake was ready. Next, I bought a great steak and Craig cooked it on a grill at the facility where he was staying. We added some salad and a potato, and he was very happy. The cake was his favorite. His only problem was that he wasn't too keen on sharing the cake with the others at the facility.

A few days later, I came by to visit my dad in the locked facility. When I was buzzed in, I saw him asleep in his chair. I walked across the room and placed my hand on his shoulder. I couldn't wake him up. I called the nurses, and they could not wake him either.

We began the long process of watching my father die. I was never close to the man who was dying so I was surprised by the sadness that consumed me. I knew if he had been able to speak, he would tell me to leave but something kept me there. Why was I crying? I guess the best explanation was that I cried for the man I never knew as my father. So many hard times, but now I clung desperately to the good times.

The vigil continued. He came close to dying so many times but would fight back again. My brother and his wife were there. My niece was there. My sister was not there. As always, my husband was there. At one point, I wondered if my dad was waiting for my sister to be there. He adored her and I am sure he needed her there. I asked my niece to call her and tell her to hurry. She lived three hours away but had not left yet. When she finally arrived, my father seemed to be breathing well. The staff told us to take a break. Craig and I got in our car and left. Only my sister was in the room with him. We didn't even get home when my cell rang. It was my sister saying Dad had died. I was right. My dad needed his daughter with him. He waited for her to arrive and then he left. It was finally over.

Sketch 15: Laugh and Cry

16

FIVE WISHES

When someone in your family suffers from a stroke or dementia, it is almost impossible to work through those feelings of loss. My parents were gone long before they died. So, just when I figured I had a handle on my grief, I went back to square one. At the time, I found it to be completely unfair and miserable. But now I wonder if God had a lesson I needed to learn. After being told that I was worthless, no one could convince me otherwise. I needed to prove to myself that I was the person who stepped forward and stood strong. There were so many days when I wanted to run away but I can honestly say that I am made of stronger stuff, and each day my father's words became harder to hear.

I will always remember the day I lost Mom. She had the stroke, and she didn't die but the woman that remained was someone I didn't know. It was hard to adjust to the fact that I would never have a conversation with my mom again. Physically, Mom sat before me, but emotionally, the woman I knew as my mother had left me. This is not to say that I didn't love this woman with my whole heart. She was warm, childlike, and a gentle spirit. But this was not the Mom I knew.

I couldn't accept the fact that I couldn't have her back. It was all too much to believe that God would "take her in pieces." I doubted everything that I had always believed. It seemed so cruel. I wondered if God was punishing me for some deed I did or didn't do. Was God punishing Mom? Was this the hell on earth that some speak of? Did you need to live through this before you could go home to Heaven?

There was one thought that haunted me every day. Maybe Mom was supposed to die the day of the stroke but because I intervened, she had to leave this earth in small pieces. If I had let her go as Dad had insisted, would she have been in the loving arms of family and friends in heaven sooner? I had resigned myself to the fact that I would never have the answer to the thoughts that crowded my days. I prayed that maybe there was one more sign that Mom might send my way, a sign that would help me go forward. Maybe just a little something so I could forgive myself and forgive those that had caused so much hurt in my life.

One night as I went through Dad's old filing cabinet, I tried to numb myself to all the memories that suffocated me. The very last folder, tucked in the back, contained the will and trust. This was nothing new. I had seen it many times. But hidden behind it was a document that Mom had filled out and had notarized. I recognized her writing. I pulled the papers from the dusty file. It was called, "Five Wishes." I had never seen this before. It had a blue cover, and from the front, it did not look to be official or important. I opened the document and began to read it. Some of it contained the wishes I already knew. Then, I turned to the page that was talking about the care she wanted if she was unable to talk for herself. I froze for a few minutes. I was terrified that this would confirm that I had not followed her last wishes. Then, I began to read the writing. It said that in case of a debilitating stroke or disease, she wanted no heroic measures. But then it said to follow the suggestion of the doctor. If the doctor said that she could get better and that there was hope, she wanted life-saving measures including a feeding tube. There it was. I had done the right thing. I had gone against my father, but I had done the right thing. Mom must have known that Dad wouldn't have her best interests at heart. *You left this for me to find.* It had been three long years of torture but there it was. I could finally say goodbye and move on because now I knew that I wasn't worthless. *I had protected you.*

If you learn anything from this story, please celebrate each day you have with parents and children. Know that we all grieve differently, and when a death takes years, those differences can damage relationships. When your frustration is bubbling over, try to replace it with compassion. Do what you need to do to face life going forward. Spend time with family and make as many precious memories as you can. Surround yourself with those that bring you love and laughter. And if that moment ever comes when you look into the eyes of a loved one and no one looks back, make sure you know their definition of no heroic measures.

EPILOGUE

The room is dark except for a small glow coming from the night light. I listen to Moses, my Golden Retriever, as he runs in his sleep. Small yips come from under the bed as he chases a tennis ball in his dreams. My husband falls asleep quickly. Normally, I would not be far behind but tonight so many thoughts flooded my mind I tiptoed out of our bedroom and into the office to write my thoughts down.

It has been six years since the journey with my parents ended. It helps to have some distance from that time. I can take a step back and see those days as lessons learned. My husband and I made a promise to ourselves that we would be prepared for whatever the future held. We started by meeting with an attorney and updating our wills. We are working on last wishes. New thoughts change those wishes all the time. To the best of our ability, we are documenting what we see the end of life should look like for us. It is not easy, and at times, it brings up some of the bad memories. But I know the consequences if we do not put things in writing. My greatest wish is that my kids go forward with as little turmoil as possible.

Each year that has gone by, I have felt a change in me. I guess you could call it a sense of calm. It has taken real work to forgive the hurt, but I don't think I will ever forget. I talk to my sister once every couple of months. I can't remember the last time I talked to my brother but so much damage was done that I never expected anything else. My dad's words still haunt me, but I find myself getting stronger every day. In fact, I have a real determination not to let those words control me ever again. I dearly miss my mom. I am not sure if it is the mom before or after the stroke that I miss the most. I constantly look for a flycatcher in hopes of a sign but nothing yet.

This was not easy for me to write. As I told you in the beginning, I grew up believing nothing was more important than family. I had no idea that mine would crumble under the stress of our parents' death. It is hard to go on and not have those people in your life. I know if you make plans before you find yourself in this situation that you can manage the rough terrain. It won't ever be easy, and you cannot plan for every twist and turn, but maybe you will have your family on the other side of the journey.

For the children that watch their parents and their grandparents travel this perilous time, learn from what you see. Find a good time where you can all sit down together and understand how the future may look for your mom and dad. If your parents are still on this journey with their own parents, you may not know the entire story yet. There is a good chance they will try to protect you from every-thing they are facing. Support your parents. No matter how good or bad it is for them, know that they will always need you. Phone calls and visits will help. Make sure they know you love them. Now, more than ever, they need their family as they lose the family they grew up with. When the day comes for you to say goodbye to your parents, you will understand how important it is to have those that you love standing beside you.

If you are in the middle of being a conservator or a caregiver, protect yourself. Don't let guilt or fear overwhelm you. Find some backup. Whether it is family or a good friend, you need that advocate to catch you when you start to fall on occasion. Let them step in to help your parents so you can walk away. Give yourself permission to protect your heart. Your parents are important, but you and your family are too. To all caregivers of a family member, I leave you with a quote from A.A. Milne that means so much to me.

If ever there is tomorrow when we're not together…
There is something you must always remember.
You are braver than you believe, stronger than you seem,
and smarter than you think.
But the most important thing is, even if we're apart.…
I'll always be with you.

APPENDIX - SKETCHES

1. KEYS

(Senior actor sitting center stage with younger actor playing his son or daughter standing beside him)

Daughter/Son: Dad, I know this is something you may not want to discuss, but I think it's time to choose a more sensible mode of transportation for you.

(Dad starts to interrupt)

Dad: Now wait …

Daughter/Son: And before you tell me the 101 reasons you are a good driver, let me explain. Your eyesight is getting bad, and I've seen how much slower your reaction time has gotten. It's not safe for you to be behind the wheel.

Senior: I just got back from the grocery store and as you can see, I'm all in one piece. I always make a point of going in the morning and never in the rain or snow.

Daughter/Son: Yes, but...

Senior: I know my eyesight isn't quite what it used to be, and I don't want to take any chances. But if I am careful, it'll be fine.

Son: What if it's not fine though, Dad? What if you get hurt or worse, hurt someone else?

Senior: I was driving long before you had a bicycle. I have never had so much as a parking ticket. I never drive at night. I only go to the grocery store and to meet the guys at the bakery for coffee and my chocolate-glazed doughnuts. Both of those places are so close that I only stay on the neighborhood streets. I am not going to discuss this with you again. I am the parent here. Not you!

Daughter/Son: Dad, do remember the other day when you were complaining about the oranges you bought at the grocery store?

Senior: What has that got to do with anything? That was an honest mistake that anyone could have made.

Daughter/Son: No, Dad, it is not. You bought lemons, Dad, not oranges. And until you asked me to taste the funny-looking oranges you couldn't tell. Why? Because your eyesight is changing.

Senior: Well, it is still good enough for me to see what you are trying to do.

Daughter/Son: What Dad? What am I trying to do?

Senior: You just want my car. I can't blame you. Buick LeSabre, best safety record on the road. Haven't had one problem with it in a decade.

Daughter/Son: Dad, I am not talking about the car's safety record, and I do not want or need your car.

(Enter a young lady named Elaine and a young man named Charlie. They sit next to the senior and as they sit, all turn to face the audience)

Friend: (to audience) Lori's been my best friend since the sixth grade. We grew up together. We both got married about the same time and we both dreamed of having lots of children. I have two boys and a girl, but Lori had trouble getting pregnant. The doctors said that the likelihood of her having children was slim to none. I'll never forget the day she came to tell me. We both cried. Life can be so unfair. But then, a couple months later, when she'd already decided to adopt, she found out she was pregnant. Unbelievable! I was so happy for her. Her pregnancy was going very well. She was the poster child for the perfect pregnant mom. She did everything she was told by the doctors. They found out she was having a little girl. They were going to call her Elizabeth after Lori's mom who died from cancer when Lori was a young girl.

Charlie: (*to audience*) I met Lori when I was in college. She knew that she was going to be a teacher from day one. She loved kids and wanted to spend her days teaching them to be good people. I, on the other hand, had no idea what I wanted to do with my life. But I knew from the moment I saw her that I loved her. I wanted to spend the rest of my life with her. She was kind, compassionate, and much smarter than I am. It took some time for me to talk her into going on our first date. But she must have seen something in me that was worth pursuing because she finally said yes.

Friend: (to audience) Lori was crazy about eating the right things and getting plenty of exercise. She was going to have a happy, healthy little girl. Lori never missed a vitamin, never missed a walk and everything was going to be perfect.

Senior: (to audience) It was the middle of the day and I was on my way to the grocery store. The sun was shining, and I was feeling happy to be out. (*pause*) I didn't see the lady in the crosswalk. I've driven this road a thousand times and I don't remember anyone ever being in that crosswalk. I panicked. I tried to stop, but it was too late. I was confused. When I snapped out of it, there was an ambulance and lots of people everywhere. I kept hearing a familiar voice. Dad, Dad are you alright?

Friend: (*to audience*) It was around 5 p.m. and I was working on dinner when my phone rang. It was Charlie, Lori's husband. He said there had been an accident. Lori was in the hospital. The baby was on its way. It was a month early so we prayed Elizabeth would be okay. I rushed to the hospital to see the new baby. The doctors said she was perfect. She was a little small, but she would be just fine.

Charlie: (*to audience*) Because of the accident, they decided to deliver the baby by C-section. I didn't know how much Lori understood. The trauma from the accident was pretty bad. Her face was badly bruised. I couldn't see much else because of the sheets hung for the C-section. I whispered in her ear that I loved her, and everything would be okay. Elizabeth was born and I held her close to Lori's face so she could see her. She had a curly mop of hair. She was pink and perfect. Lori smiled at our new daughter and then closed her eyes.

Senior: She died that night. Her name was Lori. She didn't live too far from me. I knew she was a schoolteacher. She was eight months pregnant. The baby was okay but the Mom ... it was my fault. I am so sorry. I have two daughters of my own, and I can't imagine what I would do if someone took them away. I see the Dad out with the baby, Elizabeth, in the stroller in the early evenings. I want to tell him that I didn't mean to hurt Lori. I would do anything if I could just trade places with her. If I could just go back. I should have listened. My daughter/son tried to tell me. I was afraid that by giving up my keys I would lose my independence. So now I will live the rest of my days knowing that because of me, Elizabeth will never know her mom. Oh, that sweet little girl. Please forgive me. (*tears*)

2. GENERATIONS

(One woman in her sixties or older and one young man in his 40s)

(Scene opens with son and mother standing, facing and talking to audience: 2 chairs center stage face the audience with about 6 ft in between)

Senior: My son and I have always been close. I was a stay-at-home parent, and I devoted all my time and energy to making sure he was happy. I wanted him to have the best. I was determined to raise my son to be strong and independent. The ironic part is that I don't know when his complete and total independence of me happened, but it definitely did. Being with him just wasn't comfortable anymore. I became the "have to" parent. He visited not because he wanted to but because guilt-driven duty told him he should.

Thirty-something: *(talking to audience)* I grew up in a great family. At the time, I had no idea how lucky I was. I just assumed that all families were the same, just like mine. I knew I was loved, and my parents knew I loved them. Being confident and independent was important, and they taught me that inner strength was an essential factor to becoming an adult. The ironic part is that once I achieved this confidence, I wanted my freedom. I wanted to stand on my own two feet. I didn't need my parent's guidance. And now I'm married with kids of my own.

Senior: I'm the same person that raised him. I love him so much, but suddenly he stopped calling or even answering my texts. Forget about coming by to visit. Once he got married, I became the last thing on his list.

Thirty-something: I want to be my own person. I can't be visiting my mom all the time. Work is so busy, and I have a family of my own now. I also have a great group of friends. Most days there just isn't enough time.

Both: I just wish she/he could understand! *(both sit, cross arms, and face the audience)*

Senior: Why do I always have to call him? Why can't he pick up the phone and call me?

Thirty-something: It's not my fault I'm busy. I have to earn a living. I have a lot of stress of my own. Work is so demanding I barely have time for my kids.

Senior: I never see his kids. Why even have grandkids if you can't spoil them?

Thirty-something: My kids are *very* active. They have school, sports, dance, and music lessons. They love my folks, but they don't want to hang with their grandparents a lot. They have their own life, too.

Senior: Last year, I had a health crisis. I'd been having issues on and off but suddenly it all came together. Really scary at any age but more so at my age. It was one of those times when you are reminded of your mortality.

Thirty-something: So, one day I got this call from my dad. He said that Mom's health was not the best. I felt badly, but I didn't really know that much about it. She wasn't in the hospital, and Dad didn't ask me to come, so I assumed it couldn't be too serious. I mean, after all, she'd been sick on and off before and she always handled it.

Senior: I thought for sure my son would come and see if I was okay. He called once but was out of town on business. He said something about plans with his family for the weekend. They were never at home much. There was always some trip or excursion.

Thirty-something: (*Stands and walks to Stage Left*) My husband had made plans for us to go to the beach. The kids were very excited. I couldn't change the plans at that point. I'm always traveling for work, so if I stayed home to visit my mom, I would never hear the end of it. It was important to spend some quality time with my kids.

Senior: (*Stands walks to Stage Right*) After about a week, I finally called him. I told him I missed him and that I was surprised that he hadn't come by now.

Thirty-something: About a week later, my mom called and made me feel like crap because I didn't visit. She said she needed some company or something like that. Thanks for the guilt trip, Mom!!

Both: I just wish he/she could understand (*turning away from each other*)

Senior: It didn't take long for the phone to ring this time. It was my son-in-law who said I was putting too much pressure on my son/his husband and I needed to understand that the world did not revolve around me. He thought it had something to do with them. He said I could not accept that my son was gay.

Thirty-something: Next thing I knew, my husband was on the phone yelling at my mom.

Senior: Who did he think he was? I didn't feel like I was pressuring my son. I love my son. (*Walks back to chair*) Why is it that younger folks think anyone who is a senior is homophobic? It just isn't true.

Thirty-something: I'd had enough. It was time I spoke up for myself. So, I got in my car and drove over to see my mom. I went over and over in my mind what I would say. I'd worked up quite a head of steam by the time I got there. (*Walking back to chair*)

Senior: I was so mad at my son-in-law. I knew he wasn't very fond of me, but how could my son let him talk to me like that? He knew me better than that.

Thirty-something: I walked in the door and saw my mom. (*Turns and faces mom*)

Senior: The door opened, and I saw my son. (*Turns and faces son*)

Both: This has got to stop!! (*long pause*)

Thirty-something: Then I realized this was my mom. She was older and little slower, but this was my mom. She was the lady who protected me and made me feel better when I faced all the difficult hurts in my life.

Senior: Then I saw him. It was my boy. My beautiful baby boy. He used to run to me with all his problems. He looked a little tired, but now he was all grown up. He was standing there strong and confident, just the way I raised him.

Thirty-something: I stood there staring at her, but I didn't say anything.

Senior: As I stood there looking at him, the years of his childhood played like a movie in my mind.

Thirtysomething: I had the sudden realization that the day would come when she wouldn't be standing there.

Senior: I wondered if he still loved me or if I was just another thing on his check list.

Both: I just don't understand…

(*Following statements on top of each other*)

Thirtysomething: how family works

Senior: instead of saying what's on our minds

Thirtysomething: We stay quiet and

Senior: let the moment pass

Thirtysomething: Instead of reaching out …

Senior: we just stand there and wonder what to say.

Thirtysomething: Does she know I love her? (*sits down again*)

Senior: Does he have any idea how much I love him? (*sits down again*)

Both: It wasn't supposed to be this way. (*looking out at the audience*)

3. PROUD

(*Daughter sitting on a couch playing guitar, dad enters the room, stands, and listens for a while. A woman in her 60s or older sits and watches in the shadows as sketch takes place.*)

Dad: So, what are you so focused on tonight?

Daughter: Oh, nothing.

Dad: Looks like something to me.

Daughter: I am working on a song for Open Mic Night.

Dad: It's a very interesting melody.

Daughter: (*nervous and talking quickly*) What's wrong with it? Is it bad? Maybe I shouldn't do this? I am sure I can get out of this if I call now. (*She gets up to leave*)

Dad: Stop! (*Gently*) Please give me just a minute to talk to you.

Daughter: I know Dad. I have heard it all before. I should stop focusing on music, dance, and theater. I will never get a job that makes any money in the arts. (*She continues on*)

Dad: No. I am serious. Please give me just a minute. Come on. (*Pats the couch*)

Daughter: (*Returns and flops on the couch showing some typically teenage attitude*) Okay.

Dad: (*Dad shifts and clears his throat*) Someday you will have kids of your own. (*daughter rolls eyes*) I mean if that is what you choose to do. No pressure.

Daughter: (*daughter cracks small smile*)

Dad: There are so many things people should tell you about being a parent.

Daughter: Like what?

Dad: Well, as a parent, I see myself in you. I see my smile and I see my sense of humor. I even see my love of potato chips. (*Laughs*)

Daughter: So, *that's* where that comes from.

Dad: What I am trying to say is, I see so much of me in you that I begin to believe you are just like me.

Dad: It's something all parents do. It's not fair though. Because when we try to change you or make you be just like we are, we give you all our fears, insecurities, and, in my case, a mountain of anxiety. You're not me. You're so much better. (*Pauses*) Your song is absolutely beautiful. (*Daughter has tears*) I want you to know that I'm so proud of you. I'm completely blown away by the person you've become. You're a strong and determined woman, and you'll find your own path. Please forgive me if I made you feel like your dreams weren't good enough because they aren't *my* dreams for you. I want to see you take your talent and run with it. No ... fly with it. (*Both hug*)

Daughter: Thanks, Dad.

3. Proud

Woman gets up and walks over to Center Stage

When I was a young girl, still living at home, all I ever wanted was to pursue the arts. I was pretty good, and somewhere deep inside there was this small flame flickering. I thought I could make a difference. I thought our world needed more music, dance, and storytelling. My parents didn't see it that way. They wanted me to get a degree in something that could make money and support me in case I chose to never marry. They pushed me into math and science. I did well in both, but my heart and my passion lead me in a different direction. I have so many memories of my dad telling me I wasn't good enough. I had no chance of becoming this artist that I dreamed of becoming. That small flame inside me was finally extinguished, and I went to work in a bank. I guess that would have been good for some people, but not for me. Eventually, I did marry a very nice man. Financially, I guess you could say we were secure. But I always wondered what my life could have been if someone had seen me for who I was and encouraged me to follow the path that I so dearly wanted.

So now, when I am alone and thinking of my past, I imagine who this old lady might have been with a little encouragement. What you saw today was my daydream. I see myself and my dad as I wish we could have been. I change the movie in my mind to hear him say the words I wish he had said. It might have sent me on the path I could have taken *if he* had believed in me. I think that's what every young woman needs. She needs to know that her family supports her and loves her. She needs someone to give her the freedom to fly.

4. SILENCE 1 OR 2

(*Woman on stage in chair or wheelchair. All Dorothy's lines recorded or offstage*)

Dorothy: I suffered a severe stroke. My family and friends say I look fine, but I don't feel fine. I am eighty-eight years old, but I was busy and happy. I was an RN for many years. I understood that I had a massive stroke. No one had to tell me what my future looked like. I was a mom, grandma, and a great grandma. I have been married to the same man for sixty-six years, for better or for worse. In a matter of minutes, I went from being able to communicate normally to a person who was unable to convey even the most basic words. It was a blood clot.

Since the brain damage is in the left cerebral hemisphere, which is the part of the brain that controls speech, I now have aphasia and my right side is weak and numb. It also affected my hearing. I studied about strokes as a student nurse, and always had a fear I might suffer one someday. In fact, I called my daughter, Susie, a while back and told her that if I ever had a stroke and was unable to communicate that I wanted no heroic measures. I didn't need to talk to my other children. But I was afraid that Susie, who's my youngest, wouldn't be able to let me go.

While I was in the hospital, I realized that I had serious difficulty with my speech. I felt like my life was over. The doctor said there was so much brain damage that I needed a feeding tube and months of therapy in a transitional care (TC) unit. The second day in TC, the doctor came in to ask me a question. I tried to answer. I knew the answer, but the words weren't there. He paused for a moment and walked out of the room. His lack of reaction made me feel ignored and frightened. I was devastated and horrified by his lack of care. He didn't see me as a woman fighting back from a stroke. He saw me as someone to be *warehoused* until I died.

(*Richard and Susie enter*)

Richard and Susie visit me every day. I've always been the caregiver in our marriage. My husband had no idea how nor a desire to be the person who took care of me. He sat with me, but the silence was suffocating. I couldn't speak, and it made him nervous and fretful.

Richard: I didn't want this. You know I didn't want this. (*to Susie*)

Susie: I know, Dad. But the doctor said Mom will improve every day.

Richard: Doctors just want to take your money. They don't care if there's improvement.

Dorothy: Does he think I can't hear him? I'm right here.

Susie: I'll give you two some time alone. I am going to work on my laptop out in the visitor's area.

Richard: (*He tries to say something but is uncomfortable*) It is a sunny day. (*pause*) I wish you could say something.

Dorothy: I am trying. Please believe me I am trying. I know you hate this. But I'm here.

Richard: I don't like being in the apartment alone. This is all Susie's fault. I told them to let you go. Right? That's what we agreed on.

Dorothy: Well … I am still here. So, I guess you will have to deal with life's cruel turns.

Nurse: Hello, you must be Richard. (*shakes his hand*) And this is our Dorothy. Hi, Honey. Are we feeling a little better today? (*as if talking to a child*)

Dorothy: We are not two years old. And I am not *your* Dorothy.

Nurse: Well, everything seems fine. I'll check in after Richard goes home.

Dorothy: No, wait! I'm very uncomfortable. It seems that I've lost all my dignity and now I need someone to change me out of this wet diaper. Wait. Come back.

Richard: I am going to get some coffee. (*He leaves*)

Dorothy: I would love a cup of coffee. Oh … that's right. I have a feeding tube for a while.

Susie (*returning*): Hi Mom! Where's Dad? (*pause*) I know this seems impossible right now, but it will get better.

Dorothy: (*one tear flows down her cheek*)

Susie: Don't cry, Mom. I love you so much.

Richard: (*walks back in with coffee*) What did you say to make her cry? Do you enjoy seeing her suffer?

Dorothy: No! No! Don't blame her.

Richard: (*Grabs his coat and walks out of the room*)

Susie: I am so sorry, Mom. I hope you know how much I love you. The doctor says you can come back from this. It'll be hard work, but I am here, Mom. It will be okay. (*pause*) I love you.

Dorothy: I do know. I love you too.

Susie: (*fusses over Mom*)

No heroic measures, I said. I must have had a feeling. She didn't like discussing it. We didn't get too far. I wish I could tell her that it's okay. I wrote a note to her with "Five Wishes" attached to it. I told her to follow the doctor's orders. Especially, if it was a female doctor. Female doctors are the best or they were when I was a practicing nurse. I liked the neurologist. I watched her as she examined me. I had confidence in her. As long as I can walk again and eat without this tube, I want to see my family and rock the great grandbabies. That's worth fighting for, right? It's been grueling, but I am not done yet.

I know Richard has no stomach for this. It does hurt to hear him say he wanted to let me die. I guess I should have said more to explain my thoughts and wishes. I wrote it all down. My prayer is that someday Susie will find the note tucked way back in the file cabinet.

Right now, it's time to keep fighting. I am here! Please see me. I am here!

Silence 2

Have you ever heard the expression a person can be lonely even in a crowd? It is especially true of someone who has had a stroke. Life goes on and you are there physically but emotionally you feel just out of reach. (*Block according to the words being spoken*) (*People come and go but her voice is all you hear*)

Senior: (*recording offstage*) The day is just beginning, and I would love to get up and greet the day. But as the haze of sleep fades, I remember when I get out of bed that it's up to the nurses watching after me. I am never too sure who's going to walk through the door to help me with my morning routine. Sometimes it is a familiar face and sometimes it is a person that's brand new and doesn't know me.

I've gotten used to strangers helping me with some of the most personal parts of my routine. It's taken awhile but I just try to remove myself from the situation. It was something my mom had taught me when I was young and had to face a doctor's appointment or a dentist appointment that made me sick with worry. In my mind, I would just go someplace else. I've perfected it over the years.

Next comes my breakfast. I'm always hungry every morning but if I could speak, I would tell them I would only want a piece of toast with just a little jam. A cup of coffee would be the very best. But no one has time to help me with it. If they left me with the cup of hot coffee, I could spill it and burn myself.

So many nurses, some will chat with me. I love hearing something else other than my own thoughts, but no one has put in my hearing aids, so I try to smile to acknowledge their kindness. Truth be known, the stroke has made me almost completely deaf, and no one has realized that. They think the lack of response is my stroke. I am very much aware of everyone and everything around me.

Here comes my least favorite part of the day. The physical therapist is going to help me with therapy. She leans over and greets me as if I'm three years old. Doesn't she know I was a registered nurse and that I know more about my recovery than she ever will. Stop calling me Dearie. I am not your Dearie. I am 88 years old, and I deserve some respect, not babying. Oh, brother, how do you turn this syrupy woman off?

Good! I have company! It is so nice to see a familiar face. It is even better to see Nursery Nancy leave. My daughter is talking to me but still no one has remembered my hearing aids. I can't hear a word. I know she is hoping for a response. I really hate disappointing her.

Hey! Who are you? No. Don't make her leave, we haven't even had a chance to be together. You must be the doctor. Never see much of you. I can tell you see no hope for me. You are just going through your routine visits. Just checking me off your to-do list. You should be ashamed. In my day, there was compassion and respect.

Oh, good! My daughter is still here. She is talking to me about the kids. I can see the pictures. I hope everyone is happy and healthy. Maybe my grandchildren will come and see me. I know they're busy, but I would love to see their smiles. I remember taking care of them on occasion. We would make ginger snaps and chicken and dumplings. We would all be together on Christmas Eve. Santa would come to my house. So many wonderful memories.

I must have dozed off for a little. More company?! It's Richard. Oh, good, he noticed my hearing aids were not in my ears. He is definitely mad at the nurses for not remembering I can't hear without them. I can make out a few words now. Maybe I can hear some family news.

Wow! You can feel the tension between these two. I know Richard wanted her to let me go after the stroke. But she did what she thought was best. Now who is that? Oh! That's Jim. It is nice to have friends visit. Someone offer him a chair. There we go.

I can only catch a few words, but I know the topic. Richard is telling Jim that this was not his choice. He was never good at being a caregiver. I always took care of him. We never thought it would happen this way. With all Richard's heart problems, we thought he would go first. I guess God saw it differently. I think the hardest part for me is his embarrassment. We have been so independent all of our married life. Richard never wanted to be beholden to anyone. He's mad at the world. Well, he will have to grow up. I'm going to do what I need to do to get better. He'll just have to get over himself. I love him, but right now, it's about me.

So many people here today. I've seen doctors, nurses, therapists, family, and friends. I'm never alone, yet the loneliness is unbearable. There is this invisible wall around me. I can see people and they can see me, but we live in two separate worlds. Their world is the day-to-day routine. Mine has so much silence. Wanting so badly to go home and not knowing if I ever will. Hoping the doctors and nurses see me as more than a patient. I want them to see me as someone's wife, mom, grandmother, and even great-grandmother. Know that I am loved. Know that I am doing everything within my power to get back to the world I used to live in. Please see me!

5. ISOLATION

(2 chairs and a table. Mom enters and sits placing a paper cup on a side table. Daughter enters shortly after and sits at a distance)

Mom: It is so nice that you came to visit.

Daughter: I love coming to see you, Mom. How are you doing?

Mom: I am okay, I guess. But the loneliness is really getting to me. Just having you so close is wonderful but the 6-foot social distancing makes me sad. When do you suppose I'll be able to hug you again? How long has it been?

Daughter: It has been one year and a few days.

Mom: I feel like I am wasting the time I have left. I sit in this place trying to be so careful but for what? I feel so old. *(chuckle)* At my age, tomorrow isn't certain.

Daughter: Don't say that. We just need to hang on. This is all new, and I guess we don't know if we are doing the right thing. But I love you so much that I will not take a chance with your health.

Mom: Well, if I wake up dead, I'm gonna be really pissed.

Daughter: (*chuckling*) Mom! What?

Mom: I'm saying that after all this— if I never get to hug you again or spend time with my grandkids, I will be very upset.

Daughter: I understand.

Mom: No. I don't think you do. Your life has changed. I understand that. But you still have your family close and in the same house. Your office is in your home, and you still have that distraction. It keeps you busy. *Everything* is gone for me. No more visits and lunches with friends and family. All my meals are alone in my room. I have lost three friends to COVID and I never even got to say goodbye.

Daughter: I didn't know that. I knew Evie Lou died but who else?

Mom: One week ago, Mary's husband died. I couldn't even go to her and try to comfort her. Then, just before you arrived … I heard that Connie lost her battle with this horrible disease. (*tears up*)

Daughter: Oh, Mom! I am so sorry. I know how close you were. (*daughter is restless and wants to cross the room and hug her*)

Mom: (*pulls herself together*) You know, I've stopped listening to the news. I feel like I can't believe anything they say. Between Covid and the election, I feel I can't trust anything anymore. They act as if we're ignorant and have to be told what to do. I wear a mask if I need to, and I am very careful. But at what cost?

Daughter: They are trying to protect you, Mom.

Mom: From what? Right now, I feel like I am being protected from the last bit of life I have left.

Daughter: I am so sorry, Mom. What can I do to help?

Mom: There are no answers, I guess. I'll do what Connie told me the last we talked.

Daughter: What's that?

Mom: She said, 'We have to put on our big girl panties.' And if that didn't work, she told me to drink another glass of wine.

Daughter: (*Laughter*) She was a great friend. How long was it since you two talked?

Mom: It was a year and a few days, I guess.

Daughter: You mean before Covid.

Mom: Yes.

Daughter: What had you upset before Covid?

Mom (*pause*) I was lonely and missing my family.

Daughter: No, Mom, I said *before* Covid.

Mom: I heard what you said. Oh, Honey, being lonely and missing family is not new for seniors just because of Covid. It is just because of Covid that now people recognize it as a problem.

Daughter: (*pause*) You know, you're right. Before today, I never saw it. We need to change things.

Mom: (*Smiles*) I think this is all part of the third act of life. I had never been alone before your dad died. I went from Grandma and Grandpa's house to being a wife and a mother. Maybe my generation never learned how to be alone. It's hard to learn new tricks at this stage.

Daughter: Mom, I promise, as of today I am going to try harder to visit more often.

Mom: I don't want you to feel pressured into visiting more often. I never want to feel like I am something you have to check off your list. You come visit when you want to, but never when you feel you have to. Okay?

Daughter: I am not sure I understand.

Mom: There is nothing worse for people my age than to have their family visit because they feel guilty for not coming more often. *That* kind of visit is not enjoyable for anyone.

Daughter: (*Thinking*) Is that what you and Connie were discussing when she gave you her advice?

Mom: Oh, probably! (*Smiles*) You know old people …always groaning about something. Life moves on. Drink another glass of wine? (*She raises her cup*)

Daughter: To Connie. (*Raises Diet Coke she brought with her*)

Mom: (*Picking up her paper cup*) To Connie.

Daughter: I love you, Mom.

Mom: Me too.

Lights fade.

6. FORGIVENESS

(*Couch or 2 chairs, table with papers*)

Mom: (*reading paper*) Age 91. Passed away June 29. He was preceded in death by his wife of 67 years, born on May 28, 1924. He graduated from Central High School and attended Teachers College until he enlisted in the Marine Corp where he was a pilot serving in both World War II and the Korean War.

Daughter: You okay, Mom?

Mom: I guess. (*Puts paper down*) Things have been so busy I haven't had much of a chance to talk to you about your grandpa. How are feeling about it?

Daughter: Well … okay, I guess. I feel guilty for not feeling more. Should I be crying? I feel like I should be crying.

Mom: You can feel whatever you feel. There's no right or wrong way to get through this.

Daughter: He was my grandpa, but I never really knew him. I don't think I was *his* kind of people.

Mom: What do you mean by *his* kind of people?

Daughter: I wasn't much of a party animal. Grandpa was his happiest when he had a drink in his hand and an audience.

Mom: My dad did love a party of any kind. (*Pause*) I always thought it was because his family wasn't enough for him. His friends made him the center of attention and that made him happy. As far as his drinking … he always drank too much. He never saw it as a problem. But as his daughter, I saw the uglier side of it.

Daughter: He never hurt you, did he Mom?

Mom: Well, he never hit me, if that is what you are asking. But his words hurt me almost every day. I guess I wasn't *his* kind of people either.

Daughter: Did you ever talk to him about it?

Mom: No. As a child I was too afraid. In his final years, he became delusional and well … there was no point.

Daughter: So, when everyone said Grandpa was mean because he had dementia, he was always that way and he just was unable to hide who he was as he got older.

Mom: (*Smiles*) Wow.

Daughter: What?

Mom: You are wise beyond your years. Not many people saw the real man. You did. So often people called him charming. He had a bunch of friends. They all loved the same things—boats, booze, and fishing.

Daughter: Today, I heard Uncle Bill talk about Grandpa's life as a little boy. I guess he was alone a lot. His dad didn't pay any attention to him?

Mom: All true.

Daughter: So, maybe that is why he was the way he was.

Mom: It definitely could be the reason, but it doesn't ever excuse his abusive behavior. Many people have tough times as children, but they don't take it out on their families when they're adults.

Daughter: I never looked at it that way. It's a hard thing to understand and even harder thing to forgive. (*Pauses and crosses over to hug her mom*) Well, I'm headed off to bed. Love you, Mom! Good night. (*Daughter exits*)

Mom: Good night, Sweetheart! (*pause*) (*Sitting alone and looking at pictures of her dad*) Well, Dad, your journey is over. I hope you've found some peace. I need to go forward and leave the pain and hurt behind. I need you to know some things:

I forgive you for not loving me the way the way you should.

I forgive you for calling me worthless.

I forgive you for saying you never saw me as your family.

Most of all, I forgive myself for being so angry and hurt.

Goodbye, Dad! (*pause*) I love you.

7. DEPRESSION

Monologue

(Storyteller steps out of crowd of people walking DS to tell story. People carry on discussion, laughing, etc. in pantomime, not seeing storyteller)

Depression is a true and treatable medical condition, not a normal part of aging. However, older adults are at an increased risk for experiencing depression. Depression is more than just feeling sad or blue. It causes severe symptoms that affect how you feel, think, and handle daily activities, such as sleeping, eating, and working. It is a medical condition that is treatable, like diabetes or hypertension. We know that about 80% of older adults have at least one chronic health condition, and 50% have two or more. Depression is more common in people who also have illnesses (such as heart disease or cancer) or whose function becomes limited. Depression is a real illness. It is not a sign of a person's weakness or a character flaw. You can't snap out of clinical depression.

Depression in older adults may be difficult to recognize because they may show different symptoms than younger people. For some older adults with depression, sadness is not their main symptom. They may have other, less obvious symptoms of depression, or they may not be willing to talk about their feelings. Sometimes older people who are depressed appear to feel tired, have trouble sleeping, and seem grumpy and irritable. Confusion or attention problems caused by depression can sometimes look like Alzheimer's disease or brain disorders.

Depression is a common problem among older adults, but it is NOT a normal part of aging. In fact, studies show that most older adults feel satisfied with their lives, despite having more illness and physical problems. However, important life changes that happen as we get older cause feelings of uneasiness, stress, and sadness. For instance, the death of a loved one, moving from work into retirement, or dealing with a serious illness can leave people feeling sad and anxious. After a period of adjustment, many older adults can regain their emotional balance, but others do not and may develop depression.

The hardest part of depression for me is telling my family. I have always been the parent. It feels like it's always been my job to see that everyone else is taken care of. I have always been in charge. Suddenly, I feel as if my life has no purpose. My life feels meaning-less, but I don't want my kids to see me sad and out of control. They don't want to hear that I can't sleep, that I am confused and can't remember the simplest things. What would they do if I told them I have thoughts about killing myself? I can't tell them that. So, I smile and pretend that everything is okay. After all, no one thinks the person with a wonderful wife/husband, three kids, and six grandchil-dren could have depression. What right does she/he have to be depressed? She/he should be thankful for what she/he has. At the time I need the most support, I stand here alone. I don't know how to reach out for help. You know how it is. This sort of thing makes people turn away. (*turns to talk to people as they start to leave*) I don't mean to push you away. (*to another leaving*) I am not fine, and I am not okay. (*they don't see him/her just and keep walking*)

(*People continue to leave the stage saying goodbye in pantomime and slowly leave storyteller alone.*)

The longer I live with it the worse it gets. I am invisible. Please see me. Please help me. I need someone to see through the mask I wear today. Talk to me and find me someone who can help. I'm sinking into a deep dark ocean of despair. I'm trying to reach up and grab your hand. I'm swimming towards the surface, but I keep getting pulled down deeper. Grab my hand and don't let go! I am drowning, please help me. (*the last person from the crowd returns to the stage, stops, looks at the narrator and they lock eyes ... blackout*)

8. LOYALTY

(*Dad and son sit quietly and say nothing*)

Son: How are you today Dad? You're very quiet.

Dad: I'm good. I guess. (*pause*) No, that is not true. I'm not doing well. I have a lot running through my mind.

Son: *Oh*! Do you care to share? I mean only if you want to. (*Son gets up to leave, hoping to avoid a talk*)

Dad: Do you really want to know or are you just acting like you care?

Son: I always care, Dad.

Dad: I was thinking about your mom and about her dearest wish which was to solve the turmoil between your sister and the family before she died. Mom didn't have the time we thought she would have.

Son: No one thought she would go so quickly.

Dad: Do you and your sister talk and spend time together?

Son: Yes.

Dad: Well, that is good, I guess.

Son: You guess?

Dad: No, I mean I am glad that there's a connection. I just wish she would want to spend time with me. And I really wish she would have spent time more with Mom.

Son: Well, Dad, why don't you call her and start the discussion?

Dad: It's not that easy.

Son: I think it is.

Dad: You do, do you? How old are you? How old are your kids?

Son: Dad. I am 46 years old. You know how old my kids are. They are 13 and 14.

Dad: So, you haven't had to be a parent to adult children yet.

Son: Well ... No ... But ...

Dad: But nothing. It's not easy. It can be heartbreaking. You can be surprised so often. Your mom would say it is not supposed to be this way.

Son: It can't be worse than teenagers.

Dad: I agree, teenagers are not easy. But adult children are even more difficult than teens.

Son: Sorry but you're going to have to give me an example.

Dad: Let's see! There are so many. I'll tell you about the one time your mom never forgot.

Son: Okay!

Dad: Do you remember the summer your sister rented that beautiful lake home for a family get together?

Son: Sure. That was when all the trouble started between you and Kim.

Dad: Yes. Well, we heard about the cabin much earlier in the year from Kim. She asked us if we would come. Mom said yes right away. I was not retired yet and work was a huge focus. So, I said I would have to check my travel schedule. We never heard another word about it. We were not sure of the dates but knew it would be in July.

Son: Okay ... as I remember, you guys never came.

Dad: No, we never heard another word about the vacation until your brother asked us to watch his dog for the weekend. What we found out was that she had invited the whole family but didn't ask us.

Son: Maybe it was meant to be just us kids? (*nervous*)

Dad: No, it wasn't for just you kids. She also invited your Aunt Midge and her boyfriend, a guy she'd been dating for a little over a month. Your mom and I had been having a real hard time. We'd been taking care of Mom's parents and mine. That's when your mom's health started to change. We lost all your grandparents in one year. Your mom really needed help. Both of us were working at the time. Your aunt made life hard for us. We never told you about all the nastiness, but it was bad enough that when your grandparents died, there was nothing Mom wanted more than to walk away from that and for our children to spend time with us. You had time for everyone but us. After multiple discussions with the doctor, he told Mom she needed to protect herself from the constant reminders of her sister, Midge. He said maybe we should consider relocating. But Mom wouldn't leave the area because of her kids and grandkids. She loved you guys more than she cared about her own health. Did you ever realize that?

Son: Why didn't you tell us this?

Dad: We did. You kids said you didn't want to take sides. You liked your aunt, and you didn't want to walk away from her. But what happened is that you did take sides. You sided with your aunt. So, when your sister invited them to the family week at the lake house, instead of us, your mom and I felt like you saw them as the family you wanted. They were fun, and we were disposable. The hurt was more than we could stand. I moved on and decided we would have our own life. But Mom just couldn't forget it.

Son: I don't know what to say.

Dad: Well, I do. Your mom was so crushed by you "not wanting to take sides" that she did everything in her power to keep our family together. She knew she was losing you. Do you remember how many family dinners never happened? One of you always had different plans. Again, and again, everything came before us and our family. Holidays became impossible. Other family and friends always came first with you kids. She would even call you early for Christmas, but you would tell her that you had to wait and see what others had planned first. Why did everyone come before your mom and dad? You were so concerned about not taking sides, that you couldn't see how your behavior was hurting your mom and me.

Son: Geez, Dad. I guess we didn't look at it that way.

Dad: Oh, I know you didn't. You see, I think when someone does not take sides that's the easy way out. You either love and support your parents or you don't. There is no in-between. Life is hard, and sometimes you make choices to stand and be counted. When you chose to support your aunt, you did take sides. By supporting her, you *chose* not to support us.

Son: But what about my sister?

Dad: Yup. That's a tough one. To this day, I have no idea why your sister chose to hurt us like that. Worst part is your mom will never know.

Son: I don't know what to say, Dad.

Dad: You never did. What is done is done. My plane leaves tomorrow. Do me one favor. When your children become adults and something like this happens to you. When you say to yourself—it wasn't supposed to be this way. Remember this day and what I said. Only then will you understand what it feels like to be forgotten.

(*Dad leaves son standing there.*)

(*Fade out*)

9. THE PILLBOX

Vinny—The blue pill (sleezily dressed in a tight blue suit, shirt unbuttoned with gold chains and carries a toothpick)

Ibuprofen—Walks slowly with a limp, carries a golf bag (without clubs) instead it holds a cane, a grabber, and a heating pad.

Louie the Laxative—Brown shirt and brown pants with a cape with the initials BM.

Vitamin—Dressed in shorts and a wifebeater, sweat headband, tennis shoes, and carries a towel.

Water pill—Sweatsuit, carries a glass of water and a box of Depends.

Cholesterol—Stuffed into a too tight suit and eating a giant sandwich.

Blood pressure—Yoga outfit carries a mat and a blood pressure cuff.

Melatonin—Wears jammies and carries a Teddy Bear.

Valium—Sports a '70s surfer dude outfit

9. The Pillbox

(Set consists of three big open boxes with room for 3 people in each box)

Phone ringing: *(Pharmacist answers from offstage)*. St. Mary's Pharmacy, May I help you? *(Pause)* Yes. Your prescriptions are ready. It's important that you take your pills at the correct time. I suggest you buy a pillbox; it will help you remember. Read the directions on the bottles and figure out the dose and the days. We can discuss it in more detail when you get here. *(Listens)* The blue pill is "as needed." Yes, if your doctor has prescribed it, I'm sure it's just fine. Friday. If you have any questions, please feel to discuss it with me when you get here.

(Pills come walking in with signs naming who they are. Ibuprofen is in charge. He comes limping in first. The rest of the pills, except Vinny and Louis, gather and all are chatting)

Ibuprofen: People, people, can we gather? There can be no confusion. Quickly and quietly … QUIETLY!

Valium: Chill, dude. We got this.

Ibuprofen: We have done this many times before. Why all the confusion? (pills chatter) SILENCE!!

Blood Pressure: Are we feeling anxious? Let's check the pulse, shall we?

Ibuprofen: (takes the cane out of the golf bag and shakes it at blood pressure guy) You all saw it. He is threatening me. If it weren't for me, my blood pressure would be sky high.

Valium: Dude, sit down! Breathe … *(after he breathes in and out a few times, Ibuprofen calms down)* Ok Bro, we're all good.

Ibuprofen: I will read your assignments. Please listen so you know what box is yours.

9. The Pillbox

(*Enter Vinny Viagra strutting his stuff*)

Vinny: Did someone say box? I'm here!

(*Pills all groan*)

All Chatter: (*How crude! Who invited him?*)

Melatonin: Life was a lot easier before he became necessary. A good night's sleep is hard to come by with the blue pill keeping us up.

Valium: I got that Dude! Funny stuff keeping us *up!*

(*All the pills giggle*)

Ibuprofen: People, please. Can we get back to the assignments? Okay, #1 is Vitamin. You will cover every day of the week but for now, box number one. (*Vitamin does 2 jumping jacks and leaps into the box*) Water pill, you will also cover every day of the week but for now box 1.

Vitamin: Oh, come on. Do I have to be in the same box as her again?

Ibuprofen: Yes, you do! What is the problem?

Vitamin: Have a heart man … I haven't had dry feet since water pill joined our drug list. (*Valium helps her in the box*) He smiles, and she giggles, stopping suddenly as if she tinkled a little in her panties)

Water pill: Pardon me!

Vitamin: (*hands her his towel and sighs*)

Cholesterol: (*raises his hand*) I am not as effective if I get wet. Maybe I'll be in the 2nd box.

Ibuprofen: You are such a pain!

Cholesterol: (*to Valium*) If I am not mistaken, isn't he just over the counter? Why is *he* in charge?

Valium: Don't worry, Dude, he says that to everybody. It's the arthritis (*he climbs in the 2nd box*)

Cholesterol: I just don't have the heart for this. What a pill!

Ibuprofen: Melatonin, we will put you in last place behind all the other pills every day.

Melatonin: It is hard to be last all the time.

Vinny: Well, except on Friday. When it gets dark, it's my turn (*he jumps in the box with Melatonin*) Hey Mel, how are **you** doin'?

Melatonin: Ugh! Just keep your distance. (*yawning*)

Ibuprofen: It's important that you all know your place and ... (*interrupted by Melatonin*)

Melatonin: Hands off, Vinny! (*Vinny laughs and gives her his "smolder" look*) If he touches my capsule one more time, I will time release all over him. (*They start pushing each other Valium and Blood pressure pull them apart*)

Ibuprofen: Blood Pressure, stay between Melatonin and Vinny?

Blood Pressure: I've got this. He wouldn't dare mess with me. Could be fatal! (*Blood Pressure smiles and Vinny turns away.*)

Ibuprofen: Who doesn't have a box yet! (*Vinny raises his hand*)

Vinney: Me!

(Everyone groans)

Ibuprofen: Let's put Valium in the Monday and Friday box, looks like you will be needed.

Pharmacist heard on phone: St. Mary's Pharmacy (*pause*) Yes, I can certainly add that to your order. Is your pillbox big enough for your prescriptions? (*pause*) Yes! See you soon.

Ibuprofen: Looks like we are adding to the pill box. Please hold for further instructions. (*The pillbox gang all groans.*)

(*Enter Louie Laxative striking a Superhero pose*)

Louie: I am Louie the Laxative—one in the P.M. for a BM in the A.M. (*and then flies over to the first box and gets in with the Vitamin and Water pill*)

Vitamin: (*Sniffs, makes a face like he smells something*) Okay everyone, check your shoes. Someone stepped in something. (*Everyone starts to check shoes while Vitamin has a realization*) Oh right ... never mind ... I found it. (*Pills giggle and

Water pill shifts nervously)

Louie: Real funny, muscle man!

Vitamin: Stay away from me!

(*Louie leans over to Vitamin and smiles*)

Louie: Pull my finger! (*Louie laughs while Vitamin is appalled*)

Vitamin: I am not falling for that again.

Louie: Hey, is there a place to sit down?

Vitamin: You are always looking for a stool, aren't you? (*all pills laugh*)

(*Water pill starts laughing and suddenly stops again while crossing hands over crotch.*)

Ibuprofen: Does everyone have a place and know where they should be?

Vinny: Absolutely! (*Vinny leans towards Melatonin*)

Ibuprofen: Okay that's it! Melatonin change places with Louie the Laxative!

Vinny: (*Everyone in box trying to avoid Louie*) Hey! Hey! This could really cramp my style. (*Does the drum roll pantomime*)

Pills: (*Lots of giggles … except Louie and Ibuprofen*)

Pharmacist (phone rings) St. Mary's Pharmacy, Yes, oh, the insurance expired?

Ibuprofen: You have got to be kidding! Insurance didn't go through. Everybody out!

Pills: (*Complaints heard as they leave the stage. A jumble of commotion (music up) Vinney last one out, singing to the music, "I've got that loving feeling" and bothering Melatonin as they leave*).

10. EMOTIONAL ABUSE

(*Narrator sits off to side and listens to each person share their story with the audience*)

Daughter: Dad's personality today was mean and biting. I try to visit every day, but some days are so much harder than others. The nurses tell me not to take it to heart. They say it is his dementia. But I know Dad lived his life, large and in charge. He was always first in line, then his friends, and his family followed far behind. As a young child, I remember I would do my best to avoid him when he was home. If he ever found you sitting and not actively making life better for him, you would become a target of his verbal punches. If you were busy, if you did well in school, if you made him look like the ideal parent, then the focus would be off you. If not, he had no trouble telling you how worthless you were. So, I keep asking myself why am I still here? Because no one else is.

Husband: I know Jennifer has so much on her plate right now. Between her job and caring for her parents, she has very little down time. But recently, I'm seeing a real change in her. Tears are always right at the surface. She's so quiet, removed. Our marriage feels like more of a business partnership. We just don't have the time we need to take care of us. Everything is focused on Mom, Dad, and the bottomless pit of a non-profit she works for. I am not a big talker about feelings, but I wish she could tell me what's going on.

Daughter's friend: Jen and I have been best friends for years. We both got married and had kids about the same time. It was a lifesaver having her close. As a working mom, I needed a friend to listen to me complain and understand me. But lately, she doesn't seem to have time to get together, and if we do find time for a lunch or just a visit, she isn't herself. Maybe, when I see her next week, I can get her to talk to me.

Sister: Today my husband and I drove down to see Mom and Dad. We come when we can. It is a three-hour drive, so it is not always easy. When I arrived at the senior home where Mom and Dad have been staying, my sister was there and was terribly upset. I could tell she'd been crying. She told me a little of what's been going on. Dad has verbally attacked her again and again. Dad has been that way since we were kids, so I just assumed Sis was having a bad day. I mean, you get used to it after a while. I'll just give her some time, and I'm sure she'll get over it.

Daughter: After years of being told you are worthless you begin to believe it. What is it about my Dad? He can't remember what happened last week, but he sure knows how to push my every button. He is very good at crushing my soul every time I visit. I should walk away, but Mom needs me to protect her from my dad's vicious barbs or worse. I've tried to explain how it is to friends and family but unless they face him every day, they just don't see it. People who spend only a little time with Dad say he is charming. He is a good performer when he wants to be.

Narrator: Being a caregiver is exhausting. And if one more person tells me to take care of myself, I will lose it. I wish someone, *anyone* would recognize it, and see how bad it is. I never imagined that I would become not only the main provider of my parent's appointments, clothing, food, shelter, and transportation, but also their primary source of entertainment and happiness. I keep thinking that if I just try hard enough, I can do it. But I'm juggling my work, my husband, my kids, and my grandkids while handling all the requirements of caregiving. I am tired ... just so tired.

11. THE CONSERVATOR

(Woman sitting in a chair center stage)

Voice from offstage: Please place you right hand on the Bible.

Bailiff: Do you swear to tell the truth, the whole truth, and nothing but the truth? So, help you God?

Woman: I do!

Judge: The reason for today's court proceedings is to establish the mental stability of your father, Thomas Cooper, and his ability to take care of himself. I understand, if the decision is made that your father no longer can care for himself and in fact is a danger to his wife/your mother and himself, you will become his conservator. Is that true?

Woman: Yes. It is true.

Judge: Do you know what being a conservator encompasses? You will be in charge of their healthcare and keeping track of their finances.

Woman: I understand. My brother and my attorney will help with the finances. I will see to the healthcare.

Judge: Is any of your family present today?

Woman: My husband is sitting right over there.

Judge: I am looking for any other children of your father? Your brother?

Woman: No. No one else is here.

Judge: Please tell me, to the best of your ability, what you know about your parent's health to be true?

Woman: (*Stands up and walks up to audience to tell them what she is thinking*) Look at my hands shake. Why did I ever agree to this? Well, I guess I know. I have to protect my mom. After my dad threatened her life, we had to do something. (*walks back to chair*)

Judge: Miss! Excuse me, Miss? Will you please answer the question?

Woman: My parents are presently living in two facilities. My father is in a locked facility for threatening a caregiver with a pair of scissors. My mother had a stroke and needs constant care.

Judge: How often do you visit your parents?

Woman: It depends on the week. But most often, I would say 4 to 5 times a week.

Judge: So, would you say that you have observed your father and your mother together?

Woman: Yes, I have.

Judge: Do you believe your father is mentally and physically a threat to your mother?

Woman: (*walks back to audience*) This was the part I really dread. I was raised my entire life believing nothing was more important than family. How can I sit in front of complete strangers and talk about my dad like he is a criminal? My brother and sister agreed that this was the only thing we could do to protect Mom from Dad. But where are they? Why aren't they in the courtroom? I have to protect her.

Judge: Please answer the question Miss? Do you believe your father is mentally and physically a threat to your mom?

Woman: Yes. My worries are not only physical. My dad talks of leaving and living his life somewhere else. He would desert Mom and leave her with no money for her healthcare and day-to-day expenses.

Judge: Can you give me an example of a physical threat?

Woman: (*eyeing the audience and shifting nervously*) I was visiting my mom and dad one day and my father told me he should smother my mom with a pillow and kill himself. He was mad because I had taken my mom out for lunch.

Judge: I see. I have a report here from his last home that he threatened one of the caretakers with scissors. He also called 911 to tell them he had been kidnapped and being held against his will. True?

Woman: Yes, that is true.

Judge: Your father is 89? I am assuming we are dealing with dementia, correct?

Woman: (*addresses audience once again*) I know Dad has dementia, but I also know it is not just the dementia. Dad has always had huge mood swings especially when he drank. Sometimes I was frightened as a child. I was brought up in a household where you never say anything to anyone against the family. How am I supposed to change all that and state in front of God and everyone that my life wasn't as perfect as everyone always thought it was?

Judge: I know these questions can be difficult. But you need to tell the court what is going on so we can make the correct decisions.

Woman: My father is struggling with dementia and he had some undiagnosed depression and mental illness when I was a child.

Judge: Would your attorney come up to the bench, please.

Woman: (*Addressing audience*) Why do I feel like I have committed a crime against my family? All I want is to be able to take care of my mom and keep her safe. I don't care about their finances, and I have very little knowledge of their money anyway. All I want is for them both to get the best of care.

Judge: The court does see the need for a conservator and will grant your request. However, we need at least one of your siblings present to finish the paperwork. The court will adjourn. We will reschedule two weeks from now to finalize the conservatorship. (*gavel bangs*)

Woman: (*to audience*) Wait, wait! Oh, please don't make me go through all this again. This is torture. I look at all of you as I am about to leave. You look at me with pity. Some of you don't want to get too close as if these family problems might be contagious. Some look away out of embarrassment for me. I search the crowd for a familiar face. There's my husband. He took off work just so I would not have to face this alone. There is nothing he can do to help the situation but there's comfort knowing he's here and on my side. I don't know it yet, but this is the beginning of piles of paperwork. I'll have to hire an attorney just to make sure I follow all the laws correctly. This will cause more friction with my family, but I'll do it. I'll do this for my mom. I know it is the right thing to do but it will never be easy.

12. GRIEF

(Monologue)

Your responsibility for your mom and dad can and will consume you. Is it born out of a duty or does it come from love? Well, it depends on the day.

Five months ago, my dad passed. He was the last parent out of the three parents that I felt duty and love towards. I knew in my heart that I had done everything I could possibly do for each of them. My parents had the best care and my constant attention. At the same time, I was working fifty hours a week for a small non-profit. The strain on me and my marriage was significant. I knew at the time that I was miserable and that my health was failing. Why didn't I recognize the depression and the exhaustion? As I look back on it now, I believe I was so tired, that all I could do was put one foot in front of the other. The feeling of possible failure kept me pushing forward.

The loss of multiple family members is numbing. It tears a giant gaping hole through you. The ages of the people lost makes no difference. The loss of family is suffocating. At first, the grief creates a feeling of drowning. Even with my husband so close by, I couldn't seem to reach up to him as he tried to pull me from the murky waters swirling around me. I just kept sinking lower and lower. After a while you just float. You can't get to the surface. You're aware of life around you, but it is deadened by the water overhead. You can see it and hear it, but you can't reach it. You have moments where you think you may reach the surface. It might be a moment spent with old photographs, letters, and warm memories. Then, without any warning, a huge wave washes over you. It is so big that it pushes you to the ocean floor. It holds you there as you gasp for air. Please let me go so I can breathe again. Grief washes in and washes out.

Then, you wake up one morning and you don't know how but you have reached the shore. You can see the bright sun, you hear the birds singing, and most importantly, you can feel. You feel the love from the people around you. The sweet kisses and hugs from your granddaughter. Your husband's strength and support. Months go by and an important birthday approaches and suddenly, you're back in the water again. But now, you recognize the feeling, so the panic is not as all consuming. You tell yourself to let the waves happen. Don't fight them, just float until you find yourself back in the warmth of family and friends again.

November 28th is the anniversary of my mom's birthday. It's four days away and the water is getting rough again. She is gone and her pain is now my pain. I remember the days of exhaustion. I remember my father's dismal behavior as he attacked me with his misguided anger. I wanted to get away. Now five months later, I stand alone. They are gone and with them, the anger. My job is gone as well. I just couldn't keep up the pace anymore. It had to go. Everyone has gone forward and flowed into the normal routine. I stand here waiting for some guidance or direction. Just silence surrounds me.

I wonder if my parents felt this kind of grief when their parents passed. I was never aware of it. Why don't we speak about grief? Why don't we turn to family? Well, I know for myself that I have a fear of becoming "a duty." I can already see the transition. My children are following their own paths, and we are not the choice anymore. I speak to so many women who have experienced the same loss. I guess it's the nature of passing time. Life is never what you dreamed it would be. Will I adapt? I felt I could always talk to my children in their younger years, but not as much anymore. At darker times, I wonder how much time I will spend alone? Will I go first or will my husband? At this age, death is never far from your thoughts. We are all afraid people will see us as depressed or dark. No. It is time to be honest and discuss what the future brings. Reach for the surface and grab someone's hand.

13. LILLY MAE

(Little girl sits on a small chair while reading letter to God on center stage)

Hello, my name is Lilly Mae. I am 7 years old, and I love all things magical. If there are tooth fairies, elves, Easter bunnies, and fairies surrounding you like they do me, then you will be happy too. I know if you aren't good, you won't ever have the fairies leave you special surprises in your fairy garden, and Santa will not bring you presents. But, if you are a good person and care for those around you, then most of your wishes will come true.

When I first heard about magic from Mom and in the books we read, I thought, *Well, seems simple enough! I am a pretty good kid. I do what I am told most the time. I know I am not perfect. Sometimes I can be a little naughty, but so are the adults I know.*

Now, the reason I am writing you this letter is because I need you to give me the biggest wish I have ever asked for. This is not a wish for a fairy. I need someone "higher up." I'm not even sure you can help me this time. It is not a doll and it is not a puppy. It is even bigger than a pony. I want you to help my Nana. I am sure you know her. When I was just a kid, she spent lots of time with me. She would tell me I was her special girl. We were kindred spirits. In case you don't know what that means, it means we were a lot alike. We both love animals, orange soda, and candy. I don't mean just old people candy but Skittles and Pixy Stixs ... the really good stuff. We watched movies all the time. Sometimes we would watch the same movie over and over again. Sometimes just because I wanted to and sometimes because Nana wanted to. She loved Pollyanna. Nana always said she would always be there for me. Last year, we couldn't be together. We had something called Covid happen. It made many people sick and some even went to heaven. It was especially hard on people Nana's age, so we had to stay apart. It was hard for me, but I know it made Nana cry all the time.

Right before the Covid, Nana and Pop Pop moved to Arizona. It was going to be better for their health. But the deal was that Nana could fly in a plane to see me any time she wanted or if I needed her. We knew the move was going to be really hard for us. But knowing Nana could visit me made me feel a little better but the Covid kept us apart. I talked to Nana on Facetime many times a week. She would send me lots of packages and we would laugh over the phone about all the stuffed animals she sent.

Nana and I missed each other so much, but good things happened too. The best being when Tayne and Laney joined our family. I prayed so hard for my mom to fall in love with a Prince Charming who would make her smile and laugh again. When I found out that Tayne would be like a dad and Laney would be my big sister, I couldn't believe my wish had come true. In fact, when the time comes for me to order a boyfriend like Mom did, I hope I get one just like Tayne. I thank you for hearing and giving me most of my wishes. I guess I shouldn't call them wishes like I do with the fairies.

I guess these are answered prayers. When something is really, important, I know I can count on you to hear me.

(*Letter drops to floor and sincere prayer from the child*)

My prayer this year is for me to hug my Nana and watch movies with her like we use to. I know she hasn't been very well. She stays in a place called an Assisted Living home. She needs help like I use to when she took care of me. Well, I want to be that person for her. I want to be her Nana until she gets better. I want her to be in her home again and surrounded by all the things she loves. I want her to have Pixy Stixs and Skittles except the green ones … because no one likes those. I want her to be able to watch Pollyanna just as much as she wants. But even if we can't do some of those things, I need to be with her. I know she would feel better if we could just be together. I promise I won't ever ask for another prayer … well … unless it is really important. I will sit right here and wait for your answer.

Respectfully me,

Lilly Mae

(*Lights out*)

14. MARRIAGE

(Monologue)

For better or for worse

For richer or for poorer

In sickness and in health

In good times and bad

When I agreed to this, it seemed like a no brainer. I was very young and my soon- to-be-husband was too but we were best friends and very much in love. Most didn't believe our marriage had a chance but what they didn't know was the man holding my hand loved me in a way no one ever had. I was fiercely in love with him. Nothing would ever change that. Is love always enough? Only in fairy tales I am afraid. You need to be made of strong stuff and a determination that will not allow your bond to falter.

After so many years together, our marriage is the best thing that ever happened to me. You are the face that is in my mind every morning.

The face that I carry in my dreams. It's a feeling in my heart that will never go away. You need me, and I need you.

The most difficult and challenging moments we've been through together include the death of our parents, the sometime brutal ride of being an executive director, working in healthcare, raising three wildly different children, sharing our lives with multiple dogs, guinea pigs, parakeets, and cockatiels, and our personal ups and downs. These are the moments that brought us close together. The times that took us from being individuals to being us, a couple, a team.

There were so many wonderful times. I remember when our children and grandchildren were born, the family gatherings, the vacations, the baseball games, the theater performances, the choir performances, and all our amazing friends. This has become the backdrop to our lives. This was so important to who we are. But the sad and heartbreaking days were the ones that made our long marriage possible. Funny, but I appreciate those days the most. Those are the moments when I learned the real secret to being married.

You need to be there for each other, no matter what. There is no other choice. The moment you hesitate or turn your back, your marriage is doomed. Knowing that you are there for me and I am there for you, that's what makes our marriage work. Knowing I can always count on you to come through to be my knight in shining armor. As I drift off to sleep, you reach out and hold my hand. I am safe and happy surrounded by your love.

Marriage is not always easy and yet our bond is what keeps me alive. It is the strong foundation that I rest everything on. In this world and the next, my love for you is forever.

15. LAUGH OR CRY

(*5 actors scattered around stage*)

Actor 1: My wife and I had a wonderful marriage. I always said that I was one of the lucky ones. I was sharing my life with my best friend. We had three fantastic kids and a bunch of grandkids and life was good. One day we decided to go and picnic on the North Shore. There was a little chill in the air, but we lived in Duluth, so warm days were few and far between. We threw on our jackets and headed down to the lake's edge. We loved these moments because we discussed family and work and well, anything that was on our minds. I remember her telling me this story about one of her kids that she was teaching in theater class. I loved these stories because typically they were very funny. In the middle of a sentence, my wife paused and had a strange look on her face. At first, I thought it was part of the story and I chuckled. But she stammered and gibberish was all that she could utter. I lunged forward as she fell. Sarah, are you okay? Sarah, talk to me?!

Actor 2: My wife was a Ph.D. She was exceptional in every part of her life. I don't know exactly when she started to forget things. It was gradual at first and I just thought she was tired from working too much. But soon her memory (or lack thereof) became hard to ignore. After a series of tests, we knew it was early onset dementia. How could this be? She was only in her 50s. After months of me taking care of her, the time came for me to find a safer environment where she wouldn't wander off. It was a nice neighborhood facility. It was neat and clean. I liked it because it was smaller, and I figured there was less of a chance of her being forgotten. She has no memory of me now. I visit every day, but she doesn't even react to me. Yesterday, when I went to see her, I brought her some flowers. They were her favorites, pink tulips. She wouldn't take the flowers because she said she had a boyfriend and that would be wrong. I followed her into her room. She had pillows stuffed in her bed to look like a person was sleeping there. I asked, "Is that your boyfriend." She spoke, "Yes. His name is John Travolta." It was an odd feeling. Part of me wanted to laugh but the other part was drowning in the loss of my wife.

Actor 3: After my mom's stroke, she developed a strong sweet tooth. Before this time, she hardly every liked candy. But now, it was all she asked for. Her very favorites were Snickers and Rollos. My mom was 91, so I figured if she wanted candy, then candy she would get. I kept a candy dish close to her chair so she could help herself. After all, it might be a good exercise for her fine motor skills to unwrap the small candies. One day, I arrived to find a lot of the candy was gone and Mom's mouth was covered in chocolate. So were her clothes and chair. As I got closer, it looked like she'd spit some of the candy into her lap. Her face told me she was not enjoying the candy that was still in her mouth. I made her spit the candy into a dishrag and I saw that all the wrappers and foil that had been wrapped around each individual candy. Mom had not taken off any of the wrappers. Sometimes something as simple as unwrapping a candy was forgotten with her stroke. I hadn't even considered that possibility. Mom was not too worse for the wear, but as I cleaned up the mess, she seemed embarrassed. I reassured her that it was okay. Note to self: Next time, buy candies that are not individually wrapped.

Actor 4: One of the hardest parts of staying in a senior facility for my dad was his loss of purpose. Dad worked his entire life and suddenly there was nothing for him to do. People were kind and he had whatever he wanted except a reason to exist. Boredom was definitely the enemy. Dad said he'd lived a good life but now it was time for God to take him home. He wondered out loud if God had forgotten to take him. He'd lost Mom two years before and his last close friend had recently passed away. I could see depression being a real problem. Each day it got worse. I had to find something that would help him see his worth. Then one day, I overheard the staff discussing who's turn it was to deliver the newspapers to the tenants' rooms. Everyone was busy and no one wanted to take the chore. I stopped and suggested perhaps they might ask my Dad to be the Paper Boy. To anyone else it would probably sound less than satisfying but for a 90-year-old man who was bored? Dad had an electric scooter and loved riding up and down the halls. So, the staff suggested to Dad that he would be of great help if he could deliver papers each day for them. The next day he couldn't wait to tell me about his new job. He would deliver each paper and stop and talk to anyone who wanted company. We all need to have a purpose and a reason to be.

Actor 5: After my mom's stroke, her speech was a huge frustration. She worked with therapists every day. They drove my mom crazy. They talked to her like she was child. At one point, my mom totally shut down and ignored them. They thought Mom was not making the connection, but I knew she was a retired RN who found their condescending ways to be infuriating. I tried to suggest a different tactic, but Mom wanted nothing to do with them. Mother's Day was not far off, so I decided I would find something that might get her to talk without feeling that she was back in grade school. After getting permission from the staff, I bought Mom a parakeet. He was blue and loved to sing. As I walked in the door with the handsome blue bird, I asked Mom what she thought we should name him. Without hesitation, she replied, "Petey!!" I turned towards her and smiled and said, "Petey it is." After that, Petey was her friend for everything. They watched all the Twins baseball games together. Side by side they cheered on the team. Mom's vocabulary increased each day. A lot of it was baseball related but that was fine with me.

Narrator: Watching loved ones go through the journey of aging is difficult at best. There are times when you can feel your heart breaking. However, there are times when you feel laughter bubbling over. We don't mean to seem unsympathetic. After all, our love for our parents and spouses is very strong. Sometimes emotions show through tears and that's okay, but sometimes laughter is the only thing that can get us through the day.

BONUS SKETCH - TECHNOLOGY

(*Grandma with teenage grandson by computer, Dad looking at his phone and Grandpa reading the newspaper*)

Teen: Well, your computer seems to be frozen.

Grandma: That's a relief! How long does it take to defrost?

Teen: No Grandma, it doesn't work that way. It seems like you have a bunch of extra stuff on here from when we set it up. You have at least three different viruses.

Grandma: Virus? My computer has a virus? How did that happen? It never leaves our house. I think you better check again.

Teen: No, Grandma. It's not that kind of virus. Let me see what I can do. (Teen continues working on computer)

Grandma: (*Grandpa, Teen, and Dad*) Okay! Can I get you something to eat? How about some cookies?

Craig: No thanks, Mom. We grabbed a burger on our way over.

Grandma: Oh! Well, the cookies are small. I am sure you'll have room for these. (*Grandma starts off to kitchen offstage*)

Craig: Mom! No really! Mom. Mom?!

Grandpa: (*to son as he puts down paper*) Just eat the cookies. It will make life easier for all of us.

Teen: Wow! What a mess, Dad.

Craig: (*Dad walks over to his son working on computer*) Is it fixable?

Teen: We have to fix it and fast.

Craig: What did she do?

Teen: It's not good. Look at this, Dad. (*Dad looks over his shoulder*)

Craig: (*to Grandpa*) Did you know Mom is giving money away to those preachers on TV.

Grandpa: Your mom is a good Christian and if she wants to send them a little money, I can't see how that hurts.

Craig: Geez! Dad, she's giving away thousands of dollars to evangelists and look at the amount of money to the so-called IRS, not to mention this man from India.

Grandpa: Well, the young man was an American in India and he needed to get home. I also know we owed money to the IRS.

Craig: Have you ever heard of computer scams?

Grandpa: Who would want to scam us?

Craig: Dad, seriously!? Have you ever given your bank account information to anyone?

Grandpa: Who do you think we are? I know better than that.

Teen: Ahhh, Dad ... You better ...

Craig: Quiet son, I am talking to Grandpa. What exactly did you give them?

Grandpa: Ask your Mom. I'm not sure. (*Grandpa calls for wife*) Doris? Tell our son who you are giving money to.

Grandma: (*she comes rushing in with a plate of cookies*) Here are the cookies.

Craig: (*taking one cookie*) Mom, I need to know who you're giving money to.

Grandma: Well, for Heaven's sake!

Craig: What?

Grandma: Take more than one, Honey. I made them for you.

Craig: Mom, this is serious!

Grandma: What is serious dear?

Craig: The money!

Grandma: Oh yes, that. I gave it to a young man trying to get home from India. But most of the money I gave to the church.

Craig: Your church?

Grandma: It doesn't matter what church dear. We are all God's children.

Craig: Mom, you can't do that!

Grandma: I most certainly can!

Teen: Dad. *Really?*

Craig: Just a second Charlie!

Teen: This is something you really need to see.

Craig: I have my hands full. Hang on. Mom, can you sit down, and Dad can you put the paper down.

Grandma: Okay dear, we're listening. Oh, look Bill, Craig is wearing the shirt we bought him for Christmas. He looks so handsome. Do you remember the time …?

Craig: MOM!

Grandma: You don't have to shout. I taught you better. Have you forgotten to respect your elders and honor your father and mother?

Craig: (*Sighs and looks to the heavens*) I could use some help here!!

Mom: What is it dear? Aren't you feeling well? Charlie says our computer has a virus. Maybe you got it too.

Craig: (*great frustration*) The people you are giving money to are scam artists. This is not a boy from India and this money is probably not going to the Christian greater good. They talk you into giving them money until they bleed you dry.

Grandma: I just don't think a person of God would do that.

Craig: But Mom, that is my point. This is not a person of God. This is probably a criminal from a jail cell. As long as you did not give them you bank account, we'll just say lesson learned, I guess.

Grandma: Oh no! I wouldn't do that. I just gave them my credit card number so they could take monthly payments. They were so helpful.

Craig: So, they have all your information?

Grandma: Just my credit card dear, not my bank account.

Craig: Okay. We need to cancel your credit card. Please trust me on this.

Teen: Dad … Dad … DAD!!! (*everyone turns, startled by the outburst from teen*)

Craig: Now what? (*walks over to the computer*) WHAT??

Grandma: (*Grandma follows*) Oh, that. Her name is Xanadu! Doesn't she seem like a nice girl?

Teen: Xanadu?! (*to Dad*) Please don't make me listen to this anymore. (*Teen very uncomfortable with discussion*)

Grandma: Grandpa gives her money once a week so she can go to college.

Grandpa: (*smirking over the top of paper*) Well, I thought she needed some help.

Son: With what?

Grandma: (*shrugs*) Well, she must not have much money. She always wears the same short plaid skirt every week.

Teen: Someone just shoot me now.

Grandma: First thing I think she needs is a coat or before long she will have a virus too.

Son: Come on, Charlie! (*to Grandma and Grandpa*) We have all your information at home, and I'll fix what I can. I'll call if I need any more information from you. (*Dad exits*) Please stop giving money to people you do not know. (*to Grandpa*) Especially you!

Teen: (*to grandparents*) Grandma and Grandpa don't take offense. But I never want to hear you mention Xanadu in the short plaid skirt again. Bye. (*Teen runs out the door and Grandma and Grandpa shrug*)

Grandma: Hmmm, strange!

BONUS SKETCH - AGING

Lilly Mae: (*Looking out the window and waiting for Nana and Pop Pop*)

(*Nana and Pop Pop come in the door*)

Nana: Lilly Mae, how is my special girl today?

Lilly Mae: I've been waiting for you!

Pop Pop: (*As he takes Nana's coat*) The older Nana gets, the longer it takes us to get here. (*Pop Pop smiles*)

Nana: What!? I was in the car waiting for you. The truth is, the older you get, the slower you get.

Pop Pop: That used to be a good thing. (*laughs*)

Lilly Mae: What used to be a good thing, Pop Pop?

Nana: (*throwing Pop Pop a raised eyebrow*) Never you mind. Come over here and tell me about your day.

Lilly Mae: William had trouble listening in class.

Nana: Is he naughty?

Lilly Mae: No. But he sure is funny.

Nana: What does he do?

Lilly Mae: When the teacher talks, we're supposed to mute our computers and listen quietly. William loves to unmute his.

Pop Pop: (*pauses, confused*) Times have really changed.

Lilly Mae: How has it changed?

Nana: Oh, heavens Lilly! Don't get him started!

Pop Pop: When I was a boy in school, we didn't have computers.

Lilly Mae: I'm sorry. Didn't you have enough money?

Pop Pop: No (*laughing*) Computers weren't around yet.

Lilly Mae: Wow! You really are old.

Nana: Ancient!

Pop Pop: (*joking*) That's enough out of you.

Lilly Mae: So, who's older? You or Nana?

Pop Pop: I am. I'm almost two years older.

Lilly Mae: I thought so.

Pop Pop: Really?

Lilly Mae: Yup! You look older.

Nana: (*Laughing*) That's right, Lilly! Tell him more.

Pop Pop: Why do I look older?

Lilly Mae: Nana has brown hair!

Pop Pop: Well, my hair is brown too.

Nana: I think that ship has sailed.

Lilly Mae: Pop Pop, I'm pretty sure your hair is gray.

Pop Pop: (*sarcastically*) So, ask Nana why her hair is brown? You found that in a bottle did you not, dear?

Lilly Mae: So, why don't you look in the same bottle, Pop Pop?

Pop Pop: Well, Lilly, I was once told by a much younger woman than your Nana that with my gray hair and beard, I look just like Harrison Ford.

Nana: Daughters don't count, Pop Pop.

Pop Pop: Your Nana is just mad because when we go to grocery or shopping at the mall, the people call her Honey, Sweetie, or Dearie when her hair is gray.

Nana: You will learn, Lilly Mae, that as men get old, they are thought to be, handsome and charming. But people think women just look old. They think they need to treat us like we are on the early road to dementia.

Lilly Mae: Where is dementia?

Pop Pop: (*ego showing*) I can't help that I look better with age.

Lilly Mae: Who is the Harrison guy? Is he old too? (*Pop Pop stops his strutting*)

Nana: (*laughter*) I love you, Sweetie!

Lilly Mae: If Sweetie is bad, why do you call me Sweetie?

Nana: Sweetie isn't bad for *you*. You are the most beautiful person I know.

Lilly Mae: Is it okay if I call you Sweetie too?

Nana: You can call me Sweetie any time because I love you, bunches. (*hugging Lilly*)

Pop Pop: I love you too, Lilly. (*turns to Nana*) And I love you, Sweetie.

Nana: Watch your step, Old Man! (*smiles and winks*)

(*Lights out!*)

FIVE WISHES

MY WISH FOR:

The Person I Want to Make Care Decisions for Me When I Can't

The Kind of Medical Treatment I Want or Don't Want

How Comfortable I Want to Be

How I Want People to Treat Me

What I Want My Loved Ones to Know

Print Your Name

Birthdate

FIVE WISHES®

There are many things in life that are out of our hands. This Five Wishes document gives you a way to control something very important — how you are treated if you get seriously ill. It is an easy-to-complete form that lets you say exactly what you want. Once it is filled out and properly signed, it is valid under the laws of most states.

What Is Five Wishes?

Five Wishes is the first living will (also called an advance directive) that talks about your personal, emotional, and spiritual needs as well as your medical wishes. It lets you choose the person you want to make health care decisions for you if you are not able to make them for yourself. Five Wishes lets you say exactly how you wish to be treated if you get seriously ill. It was written with the help of the nation's leading experts in end-of-life care. It's also easy to use. All you have to do is check a box, circle a direction, or write a few sentences.

How Five Wishes Can Help You And Your Family

- It lets you talk with your family, friends and doctor about how you want to be treated if you become seriously ill.

- Your family members will not have to guess what you want. It protects them if you become seriously ill, because

they won't have to make hard choices without knowing your wishes.

- You can know what your mom, dad, spouse, or friend wants. You can be there for them when they need you most. You will understand what they really want.

How Five Wishes Began

For 12 years, Jim Towey worked closely with Mother Teresa, and, for one year, he lived in a hospice she ran in Washington, DC. Inspired by this first-hand experience, Mr. Towey sought a way for patients and their families to plan ahead and to cope with serious illness. The result is Five Wishes and the response to it has been overwhelming. It has been featured on CNN and NBC's Today Show and in the pages of *Time* and *Money* magazines. Newspapers have called Five Wishes the first "living will with a heart and soul." Today, Five Wishes is available in 29 languages.

2

Who Should Use Five Wishes

Five Wishes is for anyone 18 or older — married, single, parents, adult children, and friends. More than 35 million people of all ages have already used it. Because it works so well, lawyers, doctors, hospitals and hospices, faith communities, employers, and retiree groups are handing out this document.

People who use Five Wishes find that it helps them express all that they want and provides a helpful guide to family members, friends, care givers and doctors. Most doctors and health care professionals know they need to listen to your wishes no matter how you express them.

Five Wishes In My State

Five Wishes was created with help from the American Bar Association's Commission on Law and Aging. **If you live in the District of Columbia or most states you can use Five Wishes and have the peace of mind to know that it substantially meets your state's requirements under the law.** If you live in one of six states **(Indiana, Kansas, New Hampshire, Ohio, Oregon, or Texas)** you can still use Five Wishes but may need to take an extra step. Find out more at *FiveWishes.org/states*.

How Do I Change To Five Wishes?

You may already have a living will or a durable power of attorney for health care. If you want to use Five Wishes instead, all you need to do is fill out and sign a new Five Wishes as directed. As soon as you sign it, it takes away any advance directive you had before. To make sure the right form is used, please do the following:

- Destroy all copies of your old living will or durable power of attorney for healthcare. Or you can write "revoked" in large letters across the copy you have. Tell your lawyer if he or she helped prepare those old forms for you.

- Tell your Health Care Agent, family members, and doctor that you have filled out a new Five Wishes. Make sure they know about your new wishes.

How Do I Start Using Five Wishes?

Let us help with some tips on how to start using Five Wishes and how to talk about it. Activate your Five Wishes to get these benefits at *FiveWishes.org/activate.*

3

WISH 1

**The Person I Want To Make Health Care Decisions For Me
When I Can't Make Them For Myself.**

*I*f I am no longer able to make my own health care decisions, this form names the person I choose to make these choices for me. This person will be my Health Care Agent (or other term that may be used in my state, such as proxy, representative, or surrogate). This person will make my health care choices if both of these things happen:

- *My attending or treating doctor finds I am no longer able to make health care choices.* **AND**
- *Another health care professional agrees that this is true.*

If my state has a different way of finding that I am not able to make health care choices, then my state's way should be followed.

The Person I Choose As My Health Care Agent Is:

_____   _____
First Choice Name   Phone

_____   _____
Address   City/State/Zip

If this person is not able or willing to make these choices for me, *OR* is divorced or legally separated from me, *OR* this person has died, then these people are my next choices:

_____   _____
Second Choice Name   Third Choice Name

_____   _____
Address   Address

_____   _____
City/State/Zip   City/State/Zip

_____   _____
Phone   Phone

Picking The Right Person To Be Your Health Care Agent

Choose someone who knows you very well, cares about you, and who can make difficult decisions. A spouse or family member **may not** be the best choice because they are too emotionally involved. Sometimes they **are** the best choice. You know best. Choose someone who is able to stand up for you so that your wishes are followed. Also, choose someone who is likely to be nearby so they can help when you need them. Whether you choose a spouse, family member, or friend as your Health Care Agent, make sure you talk about these wishes and be sure that this person agrees to respect and follow your wishes. Your Health Care Agent should be **at least 18 years or older** (in Colorado, 21 years or older) and should **not** be:

- Your health care provider, including the owner or operator of a health or residential or community care facility serving you.

- An employee or spouse of an employee of your health care provider.

- Serving as an agent or proxy for 10 or more people unless he or she is your spouse or close relative.

4

I understand that my Health Care Agent can make health care decisions for me. I want my Agent to be able to do the following: (**Please cross out anything you don't want your Agent to do that is listed below.**)

- Make choices for me about my medical care or services, like tests, medicine, or surgery. This care or service could be to find out what my health problem is, or how to treat it. It can also include care to keep me alive. If the treatment or care has already started, my Health Care Agent can keep it going or have it stopped.

- Interpret any instructions I have given in this form or given in other discussions, according to my Health Care Agent's understanding of my wishes and values.

- Consent to admission to an assisted living facility, hospital, hospice, or nursing home for me. My Health Care Agent can hire any kind of health care worker I may need to help me or take care of me. My Agent may also fire a health care worker, if needed.

- Make the decision to request, take away, or not give medical treatments, including artificially-provided food and water, and any other treatments to keep me alive.

- See and approve release of my medical records and personal files. If I need to sign my name to get any of these files, my Health Care Agent can sign it for me.

- Move me to another state to get the care I need or to carry out my wishes.

- Authorize or refuse to authorize any medication or procedure needed to help with pain.

- Take any legal action needed to carry out my wishes.

- Donate useable organs or tissues of mine as allowed by law.

- Apply for Medicare, Medicaid, or other programs or insurance benefits for me. My Health Care Agent can see my personal files, like bank records, to find out what is needed to fill out these forms.

- Listed below are any changes, additions, or limitations on my Health Care Agent's powers.

_____

_____

_____

_____

_____

_____

If I Change My Mind About Having A Health Care Agent, I Will

- Destroy all copies of this part of the Five Wishes form. *OR*

- Tell someone, such as my doctor or family, that I want to cancel or change my Health Care Agent. *OR*

- Write the word "Revoked" in large letters across the name of each agent whose authority I want to cancel. Sign my name on that page.

5

WISH 2

My Wish For The Kind Of Medical Treatment
I Want Or Don't Want.

I believe that my life is precious and I deserve to be treated with dignity. When the time comes that I am very sick and am not able to speak for myself, I want the following wishes, and any other directions I have given to my Health Care Agent, to be respected and followed.

What You Should Keep In Mind As My Caregiver

- I do not want to be in pain. I want to be comfortable. Wish 3 says what can be done to make me comfortable.

- I want to be offered food and fluids by mouth if it is safe for me to eat and drink. I want to be kept clean and warm.

- I do not want anything done or omitted by my doctors or nurses with the intention of taking my life.

What "Life-Support Treatment" Means To Me

Life-support treatment means any medical procedure, device, or medication to keep me alive. Life-support treatment includes: medical devices put in me to help me breathe; food and water supplied by medical device (tube feeding); cardiopulmonary resuscitation (CPR); major surgery; blood transfusions; dialysis; antibiotics; and anything else meant to keep me alive. If I wish to limit the meaning of life-support treatment because of my religious or personal beliefs, I write this limitation in the space below. I do this to make very clear what I want and under what conditions.

_____

_____

_____

_____

_____

In Case Of An Emergency

If you have a medical emergency and ambulance personnel arrive, they may look to see if you have a **Do Not Resuscitate** form or bracelet. Many states require a person to have a **Do Not Resuscitate** form filled out and signed by a doctor if you choose not to be resuscitated. This form lets ambulance personnel know that you don't want them to use life-support treatment when you are dying. Please check with your doctor to see if you need to have a **Do Not Resuscitate** form filled out.

6

*Here is the kind of medical treatment that I want or don't want in the four situations listed below. I want my Health
Care Agent, my family, my doctors and other health care providers, my friends, and all others to know these directions.*

Close To Death:

If my doctor and another health care professional both
decide that I am likely to die within a short period of
time, and life-support treatment would only delay the
moment of my death (choose *one* of the following):

❑ I want to have life-support treatment.

❑ I do not want life-support treatment. If it has been
started, I want it stopped.

❑ I want to have life-support treatment if my doctor
believes it could help. But I want my doctor to
stop giving me life-support treatment if it is not
helping my health condition or symptoms.

In A Coma And Not Expected To Wake Up Or Recover:

If my doctor and another health care professional
both decide that I am in a coma from which I am
not expected to wake up or recover, and I have brain
damage, and life-support treatment would only
delay the moment of my death (choose *one* of the
following):

❑ I want to have life-support treatment.

❑ I do not want life-support treatment. If it has been
started, I want it stopped.

❑ I want to have life-support treatment if my doctor
believes it could help. But I want my doctor to stop
giving me life-support treatment if it is not helping
my health condition or symptoms.

Permanent And Severe Brain Damage And Not Expected To Recover:

If my doctor and another health care professional both
decide that I have permanent and severe brain damage,
(for example, I can open my eyes, but I can not speak
or understand) and I am not expected to get better, and
life-support treatment would only delay the moment
of my death (choose *one* of the following):

❑ I want to have life-support treatment.

❑ I do not want life-support treatment. If it has been
started, I want it stopped.

❑ I want to have life-support treatment if my doctor
believes it could help. But I want my doctor to
stop giving me life-support treatment if it is not
helping my health condition or symptoms.

In Another Condition Under Which I Do Not Wish To Be Kept Alive:

If there is another condition under which I do not wish
to have life-support treatment, I describe it below. In
this condition, I believe that the costs and burdens of
life-support treatment are too much and not worth the
benefits to me. Therefore, in this condition, I do not
want life-support treatment. (For example, you may
write "end-stage condition." That means that your
health has gotten worse. You are not able to take care
of yourself in any way, mentally or physically. Life-
support treatment will not help you recover. Please
leave the space blank if you have no other condition
to describe.)

7

163

Five Wishes - Sample Forms

The next three wishes deal with my personal, spiritual, and emotional wishes. They are important to me. I want to be treated with dignity near the end of my life, so I would like people to do the things written in Wishes 3, 4, and 5 when they can be done. I understand that my family, my doctors and other health care providers, my friends, and others may not be able to do these things or are not required by law to do these things. I do not expect the following wishes to place new or added legal duties on my doctors or other health care providers. I also do not expect these wishes to excuse my doctor or other health care providers from giving me the proper care asked for by law.

WISH 3

My Wish For How Comfortable I Want To Be.
(Please cross out anything that you don't agree with.)

- I do not want to be in pain. I want my doctor to give me enough medicine to relieve my pain, even if that means I will be drowsy or sleep more than I would otherwise.

- If I show signs of depression, nausea, shortness of breath, or hallucinations, I want my care givers to do whatever they can to help me.

- I wish to have a cool moist cloth put on my head if I have a fever.

- I want my lips and mouth kept moist to stop dryness.

- I wish to have warm baths often. I wish to be kept fresh and clean at all times.

- I wish to be massaged with warm oils as often as I can be.

- If I am not able to control my bowel or bladder functions, I wish for my clothes and bed linens to be kept clean, and for them to be changed as soon as they can be if they have been soiled.

- I wish to have personal care like shaving, nail clipping, hair brushing, and teeth brushing, as long as they do not cause me pain or discomfort.

- I wish to have religious or spiritual readings and well-loved poems read aloud when I am near death.

- I wish to know about options for hospice care to provide medical, emotional, and spiritual care for me and my loved ones.

WISH 4

My Wish For How I Want People To Treat Me.
(Please cross out anything that you don't agree with.)

- I wish to have people with me when possible. I want someone to be with me when it seems that death may come at any time.

- I wish to have my hand held and to be talked to when possible, even if I don't seem to respond to the voice or touch of others.

- I wish to have others by my side praying for me when possible.

- I wish to have the members of my faith community told that I am sick and asked to pray for me and visit me.

- I wish to be visited by a chaplain or clergy.

- I wish to be cared for with kindness and cheerfulness, and not sadness.

- I wish to have pictures of my loved ones in my room, near my bed.

- I wish to have my favorite music played when possible until my time of death.

- I want to die in my home, if that can be done.

- I wish to be called by my name. Please call me: _____

8

WISH 5

My Wish For What I Want My Loved Ones To Know.

(Please cross out anything that you don't agree with.)

- I wish to have my family and friends know that I love them.

- I wish to be forgiven for the times I have hurt my family, friends, and others.

- I wish to have my family, friends, and others know that I forgive them for when they may have hurt me in my life.

- I wish for my family and friends to know that I do not fear death. I think it is not the end, but a new beginning for me.

- I wish for all of my family members to make peace with each other before my death, if they can.

- I wish for my family and friends to think about what I was like before I became seriously ill. I want them to remember me in this way after my death.

- I wish for my family and friends and caregivers to respect my wishes even if they don't agree with them.

- I wish for my family and friends to look at my dying as a time of personal growth for everyone, including me. This will help me live a meaningful life in my final days.

- I wish for my family and friends to get counseling if they have trouble with my death. I want memories of my life to give them joy and not sorrow.

- After my death, I would like my body to be (circle one): buried *OR* cremated.

- My body or remains should be put in the following location: _____

- The following person knows my funeral wishes: _____

If anyone asks how I want to be remembered, please say the following about me:

_____
_____

If there is to be a memorial service for me, I wish for this service to include the following (list music, songs, readings, or other specific requests that you have):

_____
_____

It is important for my health care providers to know what matters most to me. I wish for them to know the following:

_____
_____

Please use the space below for any other wishes. For example, you may want to donate any or all parts of your body when you die. You may also wish to designate a charity to receive memorial contributions. Or you may want to give instructions on what should be done with your social media or other electronic records. Please attach a separate sheet of paper if you need more space.

_____
_____ 9

Signing My Five Wishes

Please make sure you sign your Five Wishes in the presence of two witnesses.

I, _____ , ask that my family, my doctors, and other health care providers, my friends, and all others, follow my wishes as communicated by my Health Care Agent (if I have one and he or she is available), or as otherwise expressed in this form. This form becomes valid when I am unable to make decisions or speak for myself. If any part of this form cannot be legally followed, I ask that all other parts of this form be followed. I also revoke any health care advance directives I have made before.

_____   _____
Signature   Address

_____   _____
Phone   Date   Address (cont.)

Witness Statement • (2 witnesses needed):

I, the witness, declare that the person who signed or acknowledged this form (hereafter "person") is personally known to me, that he/she signed or acknowledged this [Health Care Agent and/or Living Will form(s)] in my presence, and that he/she appears to be of sound mind and under no duress, fraud, or undue influence.

I also declare that I am over 18 years of age (19 in Alabama) and am NOT:

- The individual appointed as (agent/proxy/ surrogate/patient advocate/representative) by this document or his/her successor,
- The person's health care provider, including owner or operator of a health, long-term care, or other residential or community care facility serving the person,
- An employee of the person's health care provider,
- Financially responsible for the person's health care,

- An employee of a life or health insurance provider for the person,
- Related to the person by blood, marriage, or adoption,
- A beneficiary of any legal instrument, account, or benefit plan of the person, and,
- To the best of my knowledge, a creditor of the person or entitled to any part of his/her estate under a will or codicil, by operation of law.

(Some states may have fewer rules about who may be a witness. Unless you know your state's rules, please follow the above.)

_____   _____
Signature of Witness #1   Signature of Witness #2

_____   _____
Printed Name of Witness   Printed Name of Witness

_____   _____
Address   Address

_____   _____
Phone   Phone

Notarization • Only required for residents of Missouri, North Carolina, South Carolina, and West Virginia.

If you live in *Missouri*, only your signature should be notarized. If you live in *North Carolina, South Carolina* or *West Virginia*, you should have your signature, and the signatures of your witnesses, notarized.

STATE OF_____   COUNTY OF_____

On this _____ day of _____ 20_____, the said _____
_____, and _____, known to me (or satisfactorily proven) to be the person named in the foregoing instrument and witnesses, respectively, personally appeared before me, a Notary Public, within and for the State and County aforesaid, and acknowledged that they freely and voluntarily executed the same for the purposes stated therein.

My Commission Expires: _____   _____
                                                                                  Notary Public

10

What To Do After You Complete Five Wishes

- Make sure you sign and witness the form just the way it says in the directions. Then your Five Wishes will be legal and valid.

- Talk about your wishes with your health care agent, family members, and others who care about you. Give them copies of your completed Five Wishes.

- Keep the original copy you signed in a special place in your home. Do NOT put it in a safe deposit box. Keep it nearby so that someone can find it when you need it.

- Fill out the wallet card below. Carry it with you. That way people will know where you keep your Five Wishes.

- Talk to your doctor during your next office visit. Give your doctor a copy of your Five Wishes. Make sure it is put in your medical record. Be sure your doctor understands your wishes and is willing to follow them. Ask him or her to tell other doctors who treat you to honor them.

- If you are admitted to a hospital or nursing home, take a copy of your Five Wishes with you. Ask that it be put in your medical record.

- I have given the following people copies of my completed Five Wishes:

  _____

  _____

  _____

  _____

 Activate your Five Wishes benefits at *FiveWishes.org/activate* to receive additional resources and updates.

Five Wishes is meant to help you plan for the future. It is not meant to give you legal advice. It does not try to answer all questions about anything that could come up. Every person is different, and every situation is different. Laws change from time to time. If you have a specific question or problem, talk to a medical or legal professional for advice.

Residents of MICHIGAN should complete the "Acceptance by Health Care Agent (Patient Advocate)" form
It can be downloaded at *fivewishes.org/michigan*

Residents of WISCONSIN must attach the WISCONSIN notice statement to Five Wishes.
More information and the notice statement are available at *fivewishes.org/wisconsin* or (888) 594-7437.

Residents of Institutions In CALIFORNIA, CONNECTICUT, DELAWARE, NEVADA, NEW YORK, SOUTH CAROLINA, and VERMONT Must Follow Special Witnessing Rules.
If you live in certain institutions (a nursing home, other licensed long-term care facility, a home for the developmentally disabled, or a mental health institution) in one of the states listed above, you may have to follow special "witnessing requirements" for your Five Wishes to be valid. For further information, please contact a social worker or patient advocate at your institution.

Five Wishes Wallet Card

Important Notice to Medical Personnel: I have a Five Wishes Advance Directive.	My primary care physician is:
_____ Signature	_____ Name
Please consult this document and/or my Health Care Agent in an emergency. My Agent is:	Address City/State/Zip
	Phone
_____ Name	My document is located at:
Address City/State/Zip	_____
Phone	_____

Cut Out Card, Fold and Laminate for Safekeeping

11

Here's What People Are Saying About Five Wishes

"It will be a year since my mother passed on. We knew what she wanted because she had the Five Wishes living will. When it came down to the end, my brother and I had no questions on what we needed to do. We had peace of mind."

Cheryl K.
Longwood, Florida

"I must say I love your Five Wishes. It's clear, easy to understand, and doesn't dwell on the concrete issues of medical care, but on the issues of real importance — human care. I used it for myself and my husband."

Susan W.
Flagstaff, Arizona

"I don't want my children to have to make the decisions I am having to make for my mother. I never knew that there were so many medical options to be considered. Thank you for such a sensitive and caring form. I can simply fill it out and have it on file for my children."

Diana W.
Hanover, Illinois

 **Activate your Five Wishes benefits at *FiveWishes.org/activate*
to receive additional resources and updates.**

To order or for any questions about Five Wishes:
(888) 5-WISHES   or   (888) 594-7437
www.FiveWishes.org

Five Wishes is a program of

P.O. Box 1661
Tallahassee, Florida 32302

ACKNOWLEDGMENTS

My sincere gratitude to Dr. Sandra L. Coffin MD. Thank you for your kindness and compassion. As my mom always told me women doctors are the best.

I am so grateful to Pastor Jamie Thompson. He is my friend and spiritual guide. Jamie helped me understand that I had not lost my parents. I knew exactly where they were.

My thanks to Aunt Sarah. The family member that gives me hope that everything will be ok. I will always remember sneaking out of bed as a child and going for ice cream as you told me the story of Bill and Bud the six-foot moths. I still believe!

Many thanks to Marjorie, the woman who told me, I was the sanest person she knew. You are always there to comfort, encourage, and support. I couldn't hope for a better friend.

Thanks to Cheri and Linda that listened to me during 3-hour lunches as I fought my way through the madness of being a guardian and a conservator.

A special thanks to Moses and Byrdie for reminding me I am not alone. Never underestimate the love and compassion of a dog.

Thanks to the nurses, aides, hospital workers, and the EMT's that fought for my mom and understood my dad.

Thanks to the Lakeview Hospital ER doctors who gave my mom the best of care.

I am very grateful to the therapists from Sister Kenny Institute. You told her she could walk, and she did.

Thanks to Stacey Fergelec Photography

A special thanks to Mr. Ed Towey, the Founder of Aging with Dignity. AWD is a 25 year old national non-profit inspired by Mother Teresa.

Thanks again and again Lil Barcaski. She was a patient editor that walked this new author through every step.

I would like to thank my children, Craig Jr., Charlie, and Beth for knowing their parents' definition of No Heroic Measures.

Last but not least, my sincere love and gratitude to my husband. The person who stood beside me through it all.

ABOUT THE AUTHOR

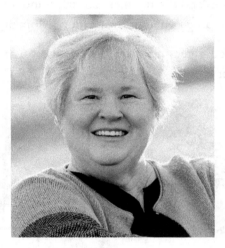

Susan Bowman Oberg

Susan is an experienced Director of live theater and Executive Director of non-profit theater arts program, targeting at risk youth. She has over twenty-five years of experience in theatrical direction, television, acting, business development, management, and coordination of special events.

Susan married her high school sweetheart at age 19 and after 47 years of marriage is still crazy about the guy. She has three fabulous and successful children and four outstanding grandchildren. She and her husband are retired now and live in Arizona with a Golden Retriever named, Moses, and a Golden Doodle named Byrdie.

Although most of her experience is in supporting and directing young people, the journey she took with her parents made her realize that the time has come for us all to discuss the third act of life. Grief is rarely discussed at any age and Susan found herself woefully unprepared to guide her parents and herself through the last stage of their life. As her struggle became unbearable, she began to journal the day-to-day issues. Her wish was to someday create a vehicle for people to open-up and discuss their thoughts and ask the right questions so families can go on after the death of Mom and Dad.

Let this story be a reminder that it is time to discuss your final wishes with your family.

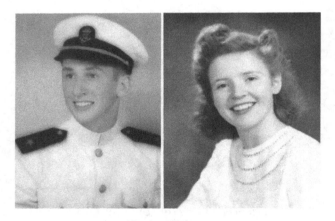

Dad and Mom